For The Health Of It!

For The Health Of It!

All the Things You Didn't Know You Wanted to Know About Medicine But Now You Do

Ali Javanbakht, M.D.

To order additional copies of this book, contact:
Xlibris Corporation
1-888-795-4274
www.Xlibris.com
Orders@Xlibris.com
84572

Contents

Book Dedication

To my loving and supportive wife, Erica, and to Zoe and Austin for being an endless source of material and inspiration and to Cricket for her tireless effort without which this book would not exist.

Foreword

δεν είχα κληθεί να γράψουν ένα πρόλογο από το βαμπίρ μυθιστόρημα «Σωκράτης», Total Eclipse της Καρδιάς. "(Του είπα ότι ποτέ δεν θα αλιεύματα επί του. Έτσι, όταν το βιβλίο του απέτυχε να συλλάβει τη φαντασία του το πολυπόθητο 12-16 ετών, νέων ανδρών και κορίτσια δημογραφικών, εγώ, ο Ιπποκράτης, δεν ατενίζω με νίκη για τέτοιες δράσεις είναι οι πλέον uη-πρέπον για έναν επιστήμονα γιατρού, όπως εγώ, ο Ιπποκράτης.)

Είναι επίσης επιτακτική ανάγκη, αγαπητέ αναγνώστη, ότι έχω διευκρινίσει μετά τη βιασύνη ότι εγώ, ο Ιπποκράτης, φέρουν ούτε σχέση ούτε φυσική ομοιότητα με Ιπποκράτη. Είναι πιο Ήμουν

αναξιόπιστα.ενημερώθηκε, από τον συγγραφέα αυτού του βιβλίου ο ίδιος, δεν λιγότερο, ότι αυτό ήταν ένα βιβλίο για την ιατρική και χιούμορ. Αυτό με γέμισε με απέραντη χαρά αφού εγώ, εγώ, ο Ιπποκράτης, είχε περάσει μεγάλο μέρος της καριέρας μου ιατρική μελετώντας την αντιμετώπιση των ανισορροπιών στις τέσσερις σωματική χιούμορ: ούρα, το αίμα, τη χολή, και τον ιδρώτα. Οχι, αυτό είναι λάθος. Ούρα, το αίμα, τη χολή, και . . . . και . . . . Ω, έλα τώρα, ο Ιπποκράτης. Ο τέταρτος χιούμορ μου πάντοτε διαφεύγει. Ας δούμε: ούρα, το αίμα, τη χολή και τα δάκρυα. Οχι, δάκρυα έχει να κάνει με την προσπάθεια που πηγαίνει σε ένα συγκεκριμένο έργο, όπως, πήρε μου, Ιπποκράτης », αίμα, ιδρώτα και δάκρυα για να υπενθυμίζουν την τέταρτη χιούμορ. Δεν είναι σάλιο. Περιττώματα δεν είναι χιούμορ.

Φλέγματος! Θυμάμαι τώρα ότι η τέταρτη χιούμορ είναι φλέγματος! Τώρα που εγώ, ο Ιπποκράτης, διευκρίνισαν τα τέσσερα χιούμορ, επιτρέψτε μου να συνεχίσει το έργο στο χέρι, με την εισαγωγή αυτού του βιβλίου.

Αφού διαβάσετε αυτό το σύνολο του όγκου, με λύπη μου να σας πληροφορήσω, αγαπητέ αναγνώστη, ότι μόνο οι αναφορές σε σωματικές χιούμορ έχει τη ήταν σπαρμένος με αυτό το βιβλίο όπως και τόσες ροδοπέταλα στο δρόμο μου όταν πάω να επισκεφθώ τον Σοφοκλή. Δεν υπάρχει σύνδεση του χιούμορ ο ένας στον άλλο, ούτε υπάρχει οποιαδήποτε αναφορά ανισορροπίες στο σύστημα χιούμορ, πολύ λιγότερο από τη διόρθωση της εν λόγω απόφασης.

αν δεν υπήρχε η υπόσχεση μου, ο Ιπποκράτης, είχε κάνει στο συγγραφέα όσον αφορά τη σύνταξη της εισαγωγής, Θα ήθελα να σας αποθαρρύνει, αγαπητέ αναγνώστη, από τη σπατάλη του πολύτιμου χρόνου σας σε αυτό. Ωστόσο, εγώ, ο Ιπποκράτης, πάντα ως στόχο την, πάνω απ 'όλα, μην κάνει κακό, και ως εκ τούτου θα απέχουν από μια τέτοια βάση και τις αρνητικές ενέργειες, ακόμη και αν αυτό το βιβλίο να αξίζει πιο δίκαια.

Ως εκ τούτου, αγαπητέ αναγνώστη, να πάει εμπρός με χαμηλώσει τις προσδοκίες και σας δεν πρέπει να είναι απογοητευμένος. Όσο για εγώ, ο Ιπποκράτης, δεν ανησυχείτε, γιατί είμαι εργασίας για το κομμάτι της δικής μου φαντασίας του για έναν νεαρό Έλληνα, ο οποίος έχει μια έμφυτη ικανότητα με τη μαγεία, αλλά αγνοεί την ικανότητά του μέχρι να αποστέλλεται σε ένα ειδικό σχολείο για να αξιοποιήσει και να ασκήσει τη δύναμή του. Είμαι η κλήση, «Ηρακλής Πατέρα." Αναζήτηση απαιτήσει, κατά τον προμηθευτή σας περγαμηνή περιφερειακό.

- Hippocrates-

For an English translation, please visit *www.healthcrap.com*

The ABCs of Vitamin D

Before you know it, spring will be upon us once again. The ways of acknowledging spring's arrival are as varied as the organisms who exercise it. Some humans celebrate spring by ignoring its coming. Bees put a little extra zest into their dances—or so I like to believe. And un-spayed or un-neutered neighborhood cats start doing their version of 'The Marriage of Figaro' on the fence every night—except they use the feline pronunciation of 'Figaro', 'Mrrrooowwwwr.'

On a molecular level, our bodies acknowledge the increased hours of sunshine by producing more vitamin D. This has been a good year for vitamin D. It has been getting a lot of attention in the media and many are calling for people to consume more of it, making now the perfect time to buy vitamin D stock—stock meaning broth, not a piece of a company. Although if vitamin D ever incorporates itself and goes public, dump Microsoft and buy some.

Human skin has the ability to make vitamin D when exposed to sunlight. Human skin also has the ability to become cancerous when exposed to sunlight. So what is a health conscious human to do? Fortunately, the answer is muddled in ambiguity so everyone has an opportunity to be right. There are no set guidelines for how much sun exposure is needed to produce adequate vitamin D. The amount of vitamin D made by the skin varies greatly by latitude, time of year, skin tone, and use of sun protection.

Since sun exposure can be such a double-edged sword, how about food as a source of vitamin D? Since vitamin D is a fat-soluble vitamin, it likes to hide in fatty foods. Cod liver oil is loaded with vitamin D. Since no one has touched the stuff since 1932, other foods may be considered. Fatty fish, such as salmon or tuna, contains some vitamin D. All milk in the United States is fortified with vitamin D. And egg yolk has a small amount of vitamin D. Again, there are no clear guidelines as to the recommended intake of these foods. Since all these foods are fatty (except non-fat milk), one must be careful not to undo the benefits of vitamin D by over-consuming fats that could cause obesity and heart disease.

The next option in vitamin D supplementation is vitamin D supplements. It is generally recommended that menopausal women take vitamin D supplements. The American Academy of Pediatrics recommends that breast-fed infants receive vitamin D supplementation also. So where does that leave the rest of us? Again, there are no clear guidelines. Until now, the recommendations for vitamin D intake had been 400 International Units (IU) for adults under 60 and 600 IU for adults over 60. But some are suggesting that, based on new research, those guidelines should be spring-cleaned along with the hairy spaghetti in the 'fridge. While the optimum intake of vitamin D hasn't been established yet, intake of up to 2000 IU per day for healthy people over one year of age is generally regarded as safe.

The one thing most experts do agree on is the ideal blood levels for vitamin D. The blood test can tell if our level is normal, borderline, or low. There is also further agreement that people with low or borderline blood levels need extra supplementation. Beyond that, the concensus breaks down once again like a child facing a spoonful of cod liver oil.

So as we celebrate this spring, let us continue to make healthier choices. Being active outdoors has many benefits besides potentially increasing vitamin D levels. And it is always prudent to use sun protection to its fullest. Enjoying a serving of salmon on a fresh spring evening can be quite enjoyable and healthy regardless of its vitamin D level. And as for supplements, we can at least take comfort in knowing that we're all equally in the dark on that one on these bright spring days.

A Case of Mistaken Identity

Imagine that you have just purchased and installed the Mega-Arson 5000 Home Smoke Detector/Extinguisher Unit. This system will detect smoke and automatically extinguish it. In fact, it is so advanced that it can differentiate between structural and chemical fires and disburse water or CO_2 appropriately. Now imagine that every time you boil water to make pasta, the unit mistakes the steam for chemical smoke. Next thing you know, you're standing hip deep in foam. Put on some dance music and put a burly guy out front, and young, well-dressed people will line up around the block to pay $20 just to get in!

Our body's immune system is somewhat similar to the Mega Arson 5000. We have two pathways of response to invasion by foreign substances: One is for fighting bacteria and viruses and another is for fighting parasites. (Keep in mind that this is a gross simplification of an intensely complicated system that, after decades of study, we have only the faintest notion of its workings.)

As with our temperamental Arson 5000 unit, our bodies can react to things that are not attacks on the body and trigger an immune response. Such is the case with allergies: Harmless substances, such as pollen, are mistaken by the body's immune system as invading parasites and trigger the immune response for parasites. This involves swelling of nose passages, increasing mucus, and sneezing to push those wormies back to whichever dark corner from which they crawled out.

With our near record rainfall this past season, we have not only been blessed with flash floods and high poison oak counts, we also have high levels of pollen, bringing out a whole new crop of allergy sufferers.

With the shelves upon shelves of over-the-counter allergy medication and a barrage of television commercials for allergy products, how is the average allergy sufferer to know where to start?

Fret not. That's where your friendly neighborhood primary care provider comes in. Armed with years of theoretical, practical, and at times personal experience, she/he will help guide you through the labyrinth that is allergy treatment.

Let's briefly review some of the major players.

In the north corner: the antihistamine. This pill blocks the effect of histamine, the ultimate body chemical that causes allergy symptoms. Imagine your allergy response as the most elaborate trap Wile E. Coyote ever set for the Road Runner. Histamine is the anvil that's supposed to drop on the Road Runner. So whether Wile E. Coyote starts the sequence by jumping on the see-saw which lifts the candle, that heats the water whose steam turns a mill which cranks a pulley that turns the fan that blows a kite holding a knife toward the rope that holds the anvil or Wile E. Coyote starts the sequence by dropping a boulder on the see-saw, the end result is the same: The anvil drops.

So, whether the allergic process is triggered by indoor/outdoor, plant/animal, or earthly/alien allergens, the end result is the release of histamine. Therefore blocking histamine will help treat the allergic reaction regardless of the trigger.

Antihistamines come in many different shapes, sizes, colors, and consistencies. Most famous are diphenhydramine (Benadryl) and loratadine (Claritin). Loratadine is a once-a-day medication and doesn't make people drowsy. Diphenhydramine is slightly more powerful but does make people drowsy. In fact, it is illegal to drive while under the influence of diphenhydramine.

In the south corner: the steroid sprays. No, not the ones that make you buff. They are similar to cortisone or prednisone but since they're sprayed into the nose, they only work in the nose and leave the rest of the body alone. So for those looking to gain weight, thin out their bones and raise their blood pressure and blood sugar, these simply won't do. The steroid sprays are by far the most effective agent that we have. They are the virtual 007 of allergy medications. They are smooth, slick, and sometimes smell nice.

So rise up fellow allergy sufferers. We shall suffer no more. Get out there and show those pollens who's boss. Sure they may outnumber us, but we're smarterer.

ADD/ADHD

I'm sure I've said this before, but it bears repeating: the brain is an amazing organ. And back-to-school is a prime example of that. Young brains across the nation start to rev up their academic parts which have been idle all summer while trying to retain the Hanna Montana song catalog and text message fingering patterns. Fortunately, the bicycle-riding part is safe and sound.

Once back in school, the brain has to start handling large streams of information that pour in over long periods of time. In order to retain the information, the attention-sustaining part of the brain must also work well.

Yes, the brain has a special part designed to keep attention focused on a certain task and to block out distractions. When this part of the brain doesn't communicate well with the other parts, the brain gets easily distracted and has difficulty staying on task.

Given that it's also model year-end clearance time at your local car dealer, we can make the analogy to a car: The brain is like a top-of-the-line sports car with 450 horsepower, hydrogen cell technology, cup holders, satellite television and microwave. It can hug the tightest turns and deliver soup in a hurricane without spilling a drop. But if the steering system isn't working well, it would be difficult to control the vehicle in inclement weather and to negotiate turns (navigational negotiation, not nuclear).

This is called ADD or ADHD. ADD stands for Attention Deficit Disorder. ADHD stands for Attention Deficit Hyperactivity Disorder (not Attention Deficit in High Definition.) The difference between them, as the names suggest, is that one has hyperactivity as part of it and the other does not.

People with ADD are sometimes called 'daydreamers', since they can sit still in one place, but their minds wander and the next thing they know, they've missed a good part of the lecture. With ADHD, people have a difficult time physically sitting through a class, never mind being able to keep their mind focused on the topic.

But people who have ADD and ADHD have perfectly well-functioning brains. The creative, logical, analytical, social, and emotional parts all run well. It's just that the attention-sustaining part doesn't communicate well with the other parts of the brain. To continue with the car analogy: just because the steering doesn't engage, it doesn't mean that the car's horsepower is lessened or that the cup holders stop working.

Fortunately, there are medications that can act as steering boosters for brains with ADD/ADHD. Medications in this family tend to be stimulants like methylhenidate (Ritalin) and dextroamphetamine (Dexedrine). I sometimes wonder what the medical community's reaction was when this type of treatment was first proposed. After all, what sense does it make to give a child that's already hyperactive a stimulant? We might as well use gasoline to put out fires or use steak to ward off wolves.

But as it turns out, these medications do help. The reason is that while these medications can stimulate the entire brain, in people with ADD/ADHD, they help the steering mechanism of the brain engage better. The effect is that the brain as a unit is able to keep attention longer and hyperactivity actually diminishes. People with ADD/ADHD who take medication appropriately tend to allow the other parts of their brain to achieve fuller potential.

So as we all use our state-of-the-art GPS navigation systems (voiced by Catherine Zeta Jones) to push forth on our quest for knowledge, may the steering column continue to do its job. And if it should falter, we know that there are repair shops available that can help improve performance. And the best part is that our brains come with a lifetime warranty. See your authorized dealer for details.

Afrin: The Perfect Drug

Pop Quiz, you SAT hopefuls/expatriates!

Oxymetazoline is to nasal congestion as:

- a.) wood is to fire
- b.) prudence is to conflagration
- c.) farinaceous is to bellicosity
- d.) a and b
- e.) neither c nor a, but including b
- f.) none of the above: oxymetazoline is not even a word.

I don't know what the real answer is which should give you a clue as to my verbal SAT scores. I'm grateful for the 200 points I got for signing my name. But if I had to conjecture, which I'm assuming means 'guess', I would go with 'a'.

Perhaps the whole thing would make more sense if we were to use oxymetazoline's alias—Afrin. Now it's all coming together.

Oxymetazoline (let's use 'oxy-m' for short) is well known for its decongestant properties. Speaking from personal experience, it is almost too powerful. I'm not sure if the human nostril was ever meant to be that 'open'.

But there's a darker side to this drug. Some people know that using Afrin for more than three days can result in addiction! Or, shall we say, dependence. What's the difference? Actually, plenty.

I don't know about you, but I have yet to be propositioned by someone in a dark alley to buy Afrin. (What I *have* been propositioned for involves body piercings and lots of whipped cream.) I have yet to hear of a police crackdown on an underground Afrin-smuggling network. I don't know of anyone who has lost their job, family, and/or money to Afrin. I have never heard of any AUA (Afrin Users Anonymous) meetings.

I have, however, known plenty of people who, upon exceeding the recommended three days' usage have needed to use it more and more, otherwise they 'can't breathe'.

That is dependence: needing more and more of a drug to get the same effect. The same thing can happen with alcohol, heroin, and morphine, but those substances are considered addictive. So how is oxy-m different?

Addictive substances tend to 'tickle' our brain's pleasure center. That is why people will forego everything they hold dear to acquire the drug. The pleasure sensation is so intense that it starts to take priority over food, drink, and social and family obligations.

Oxy-m, as pleasurable as it may be to some, does not affect the pleasure center of the brain. The only 'buzz' you get is the rush of fresh air—or smog for our friends down in Los Angeles—through open airways.

Then why the three-day warning? It's because of the 'tolerance'.

Oxy-m is a nasal decongestant—it narrows the blood vessels on the inside of your nose, which reduces the swelling of the walls of the nose. This opens your nostrils. Home remedy tip: That's why it can also help stop nosebleeds. After a few days' use, the blood vessels in the nose get so used to having the drug around, that when it's *not* around, they get more widely open than ever, leading to more swelling of the lining of the nose, which makes for an ever-so-congested pair of nostrils.

Frankly, it's pure genius. A drug that over time causes the same symptoms it was initially meant to treat! Give the Nobel Prize for business ingenuity to that lab! And if there isn't a Nobel Prize for business ingenuity, I say we make one just so we can give it to them. It's like a humidifier that actually dries up the air when not in use. Or hair gel that makes hair extra frizzy as it wears off. We could launch a whole line of self-use-propagating products!

So now we see that oxy-m can indeed be wood to the fire of nasal congestion through 'tolerance'. Didn't think I could bring it back around, did you?

Antibiotics and Cold— or Just Say No

The cold and flu season will be upon us sooner than you can say, 'Don't cough on me!' Like every other year, scores of sore throats, runny noses, coughs, and chest congestions will make their way to their health care providers seeking relief. But with all the might a fury of modern medicine, we still cannot cure the common cold. We can clear noses with decongestants. We can soothe coughs with cough syrup. We can relieve sore throats with analgesics. But we cannot rid the body of the cold or flu virus. Fortunately, the body does a very good job of this on its own.

Yet many people still harbor the misconception that antibiotics will cure their cold, or that it will keep it from getting worse, or it will prevent it from turning into pneumonia or sinusitis. In reality, the only thing antibiotics will do for a viral illness is to set the stage for resistant bugs.

Picture your body as a pristine garden. Viruses are like weeds growing in the garden and bacteria are like gophers digging tunnels and eating the roots of your favorite rose bush. As a new home owner, I have a whole new appreciation for this sort of thing. Taking antibiotics for a viral infection is like trying to kill off weeds with gopher poison. Now imagine if every time you put gopher poison on the weeds, the gophers got stronger and more resistant to the poison. Soon, you'd have super gophers ruining your garden and all the poison in the world couldn't stop them. All you could do is sit by helplessly and watch your roses fall one by one.

This is the situation in which we're finding ourselves today. Bacteria have become more and more resistant due to the misuse of antibiotics. We now have certified 'super bugs' that cannot be killed by any antibiotic we have.

So how does one tell if one has a viral or bacterial infection? It's quite simple. A degree from an accredited medical, PA, or NP school and enough clinical experience with cases usually does the trick. Fortunately for us all, there are plenty of qualified, astute, and caring healthcare providers out there ready to help. All it requires on the part of the patient is trust. Trusting that your provider will provide antibiotics if appropriate. Trusting that if your provider is using 10 precious managed-care-time-crunched minutes to explain why antibiotics are not necessary when writing a prescription takes less than one minute, they truly have your best interests at heart. So the next time your provider doesn't give you antibiotics for a cold, give them a warm smile, a firm handshake, and thank them for helping keep your garden gopher-free.

Antioxidants

Anti-cents

The jig is up. The sledge-hammer of truth hath made crumble the grandiose palace of health supplements. Or at least there's a large stain on their marble façade.

A recent article in *Lancet*, which is the medical equivalent of *Newsweek* but with fewer pictures, talked about the effect of antioxidants (vitamin E and beta-carotene) on the prevention of heart attacks. Their study was a meta-analysis, which means they took data from other studies and put them all in one pot to make it a bigger study. It's a way of doing research with a lot of people without doing research with a lot of people. All in all, 130,000 patients had participated in studies with beta-carotene, and 81,000 patients in studies with vitamin E. The researchers looked at the effect of these antioxidants in preventing a first, or repeat, heart attack.

When all was said and done, the antioxidant group had the same number of heart attacks as the non-antioxidant group. The only difference being in their respective bank accounts. (That last part was my own speculation.)

It's about time somebody looked to see if all the claims made by dietary supplement manufacturers hold any truth. It's actually quite a nice set-up: Process some naturally occurring substances, make it into a pill, put in a bottle, and tell the public it helps improve *(insert malady here)*. Package and market it as a 'food item' and thus be free from the scrutiny of the FDA, or the burden of scientific proof. No wonder it's a multi-billion-dollar-a-year industry.

But now you can scratch beta-carotene and vitamin E off your GNC list, at least until they come up with a new claim for its effectiveness. Take the extra money and give it to charity.

Hopefully, we haven't seen the last of such investigative research into the claims of dietary supplements.

Most people use these products as a 'natural' way of staying healthy. I fully commend anyone who takes an interest in their health and wants to do the right thing. But consider this: how many things in nature come in pill form? If a plant gets processed, washed, ground, mixed with adhesives, compressed into a pill form, and placed in a bottle, how 'natural' is it? Most of us are better off going to the farmers' market. (Check your local listings for time and place.) Just the walk there will probably do more good than all the pills in a supplement store.

Asleep, But Not Sneezing

There are many pleasant things about living in Santa Barbara: abundant sunshine, beautiful sandy beaches, and the Spearmint Rhino. There are also some not so pleasant things about living in Santa Barbara: slow traffic on the 101 South at Milpas, unaffordable real estate, and the Spearmint Rhino.

To the list of unpleasant things, we can add 'histamine'. Histamine is what brings about allergies. When an allergen (a substance that can trigger an allergic reaction, like pollen, dust, etc.) enters an orifice (specifically the ears, eyes, nose, and mouth), histamine is released. The result is itching, watery eyes, a stuffy, runny nose, and sneezing.

While we may not have quick, personalized fixes for traffic or expensive housing, we do have some for histamine. They're called 'anti-histamines'. (Although, I like to think of them as 'pro-itch-relief'. 'Anti-histamine' is so negative.)

If we were contestants on the Family Feud and the question was 'Name an anti-histamine', we would all slam our hands on the buzzer and blurt out, 'Diphenhydramine!' and then quickly look away to avoid getting smooched by the host. Diphenhydramine is best known by its brand name, Benadryl.

Most people know that diphenhydramine is a strong allergy medication. Most people also know that diphenhydramine can make people sleepy. That is why it is the active ingredient in virtually all over-the-counter sleeping aids, including Nyquil and Tylenol PM.

What most people don't realize is that, like alcohol, regardless of how 'awake' someone feels after taking diphenhydramine, it still slows down reaction times. In fact, because of this effect, it is illegal to drive while under the influence of diphenhydramine. I don't get the feeling that this is a very strictly enforced law—at least not until we have a good breath, blood, or urine test to detect its levels. But once we do, I think the Santa Barbara Police Department should be very wary of anyone they pull over who is not talking in a nasally voice.

But there is another option for itch control. It's once a day and it's non-drowsy. It goes by the name loratadine, aka Claritin. Loratadine can do all the things diphenhydramine can, without the sedation and slowing. It's generic so the price is reasonable and it's over-the-counter, which makes it more readily accessible.

But wait! There's more! Just as we were getting comfortable with this two-man race, in comes cetirizine, aka Zyrtec. It, too, is a once-a-day allergy medication and I'm sure there will be an advertising blitz to help sell it. However, cetirizine has the same sedation and slowing side effect that diphenhydramine does. I don't think we have a law against driving after taking it. Perhaps someone could bring it up at the next City Council meeting.

So the next time we try to decipher medication labels through the allergic haze covering our eyes, we can be more aware of our options. Not only can we get our allergies under better control, but we'll have the option of being awake enough to thoroughly enjoy all the perfections and imperfections of this wonderful little town—juice bars and all.

Attack of the Killer

Antidepressants!

A giant Prozac pill rolls across Downtown, USA, crushing cars and crumbling buildings. People run around frantically. A woman runs up to the camera, hands on her cheeks, and screams, 'If only we knew'!

Cut to a farm house. The farmer in the field squints towards the horizon. A cloud of dust has gathered and seems to be getting bigger. His expression changes from curiosity to horror. He runs towards the house, yelling at his little girl sitting on the porch playing with a home-made doll, 'Get inside!' The girl freezes, dumbfounded. The father continues to run towards her as the cloud gets closer and closer. He grabs his daughter, runs inside, and slams the door shut just as the house gets covered in little Zoloft pills.

If I had the budget for a B movie and were looking to capitalize on the recent FDA warning, these are just a few of the scenarios I'd imagine. I'd also be sure to cast Kate Hudson in *any* role.

I don't know how this is being portrayed in the lay media, but I'm sure it will cause some concern among the millions of patients on antidepressants and their loved ones. I can just picture Paul Moyer of Channel 4 News coming on during a commercial break, his face stern yet bearing that smirk that makes you wonder, and say, 'Could your antidepressants be killing you? Find out at 11'.

The actual FDA warning is not nearly as exciting as any of these:

> 'FDA has been closely reviewing the results of antidepressant studies in children, since June 2003, after an initial report on studies with paroxetine (Paxil), and subsequent *reports on studies* of other drugs, *appeared* to *suggest* an *increased risk* of *suicidal thoughts* and *actions* in the children given antidepressants. There were no suicides in any of the trials.' [Emphasis mine.]

The report goes on to say:

> '... it was unclear whether certain behaviors reported in these studies represented actual suicide attempts, or other self-injurious behavior that was not suicide-related.'

Seems like we had more evidence of Weapons of Mass Destruction in Iraq.

In the same light, I'd like to put out my own advisory: I'm sure that some reports of studies will appear to suggest that in the year 2003, there were more car accidents than in the year 1993. Therefore, I advise everyone to use caution while driving.

The initial study mentioned was done in the United Kingdom on children taking paroxetine (Paxil). Some of the children showed violent behavior towards themselves. The more important questions that remain unanswered are: Were these violent acts a result of suicidal thought? If the children were *not* on Paxil, would they still exhibit such behaviors? Would their behavior have been *worse* if they were not on Paxil at the time?

People are prescribed antidepressants because they have depression. People with depression can have suicidal thoughts. People are started on antidepressants, or have the dose increased because the depression is not under control. People with uncontrolled depression are at a higher risk of having suicidal thoughts. So is it the medication that is making some people have suicidal thoughts, or is it the disease? Hopefully, the FDA won't cause more problems than it solves by people stopping their antidepressants based on incomplete information. I'm sure then, we'd certainly see a rise in suicidal thoughts and behaviors. Fortunately, most people have enough common sense to consult their doctor before stopping their medications.

So the gist of the advisory is to be cautious when starting or adjusting the dose of an antidepressant. It's not very exciting, as well it shouldn't be. It's just common sense. So continue taking your antidepressants, and drive safely.

The Audacity of Grope

Dear Blue Cross of California,

What's this I hear about a letter going out to other doctors? Not only do I not get one, but I find out about it through patients and the internet! It seems like the whole world knew about these letters before me. The least you could have done was to call me—or email (you do still have a computer, right)? Heck, I'd even settle for a text message, but this . . . .

What happened to our relationship? I put my mistrust in you. Our entire relationship was built on mistrust. You maximize profits while I try to do my job within your restrictions.

A friend of mine knows someone who used to date the janitor of one of these 'other' doctors and he managed to get me a copy. (I thought *I* was your 'Dear Provider'.) In it, you asked these special 'other' doctors to inform you of patients who have illnesses that they did not list on their application for health insurance. You would, in turn, use this as justification to cancel their coverage. The letter outraged those special doctors and now you have a 'cease and desist' order from the American Medical Association (AMA), not to mention the 'Stand down, soldier!' order that's pending from the Pentagon and the 'Don't call us, we'll call you' request from the Casting Society of America. Even the 'Governator' (California Governor Arnold Schwarzenegger, previously the Terminator, for those of you not living in California) has raised his voice in protest.

If you had sent this letter to me ahead of time, I could have told you about the following observations:

First, if the plan had worked, you would probably be able to cancel the coverage of a few patients. But people would soon catch on and would simply stop going to their doctors for treatment of their health conditions. While that may sound like a good quarterly profit booster, in the long run, these patients would develop complications of their illnesses which would lead to more emergency room visits and hospitalizations—which is the nightmare of managed care. Don't even get me started on the ethical implications of risking people's health. Furthermore, it wouldn't exactly make new patients rush to sign a policy with you.

Second, doctors wouldn't do this kind of thing even if it were requested by someone they like.

Third, I must question the timing of a highly unpopular move that, to most observers, would only serve to antagonize patients and the medical industry right around the build-up to a presidential election where healthcare, and specifically the existence of the managed care system as we know it, is one of the top issues. And if you can write a sentence that long, we both need to take remedial English.

I'm sure the person who came up with this idea and the other person in the board room who said, 'Hey, that's a *great* idea! Our profits were only in the low billions last year!', now have their résumés posted online at *monster.com, careerbuilder.com* and *youknowtheguywhocameupwiththebluc rossi-deathatwasme.com.*

So those are my thoughts. And by the way, all those times I said I didn't mind calling to get authorization for patients—I lied! I don't like it at all. And your hold times are actually longer than all the other insurance companies. And your logo is dull. So there!

I must go now. I have a date with myself to watch 'Love Story', sing aloud to Gloria Gaynor's 'I Will Survive', and binge on refined carbohydrates.

If you care to write back, you know where to reach me. But know that it'll take a lot to win back my mistrust.

The Aural Trilogy

Summer means many things to many people. For some, it is a time to indulge in confections (especially the cold, creamy kind). For others, it is a time for vacation. For *the* 'Others', it's time to take a break from messing with the minds of us and the survivors of Oceanic Flight 815 so the writers can think of more confusing storylines to throw at us in the fall.

For most people, summertime means some type of contact with water beyond the ritual of scheduled body cleansing. People go to beaches, lakes, rivers, and (if you live in the 'urban jungle' of a soft drink commercial) blown-out fire hydrants. They immerse their bodies in water using various means and devices. They bring home with them sand, salty skin, some unwanted intestinal guests, and the occasional 'swimmer's ear'.

'Swimmer's Ear' is like 'Tennis Elbow' or 'Biathlon Thumb': One does not have to be a participant in the respective sport to suffer from the ailment.

In fact, the 'Ailments Named After Sports' industry is a budding one and now is the time to jump on the band wagon. It's very simple: pick a body part and a sport. That's all. The two don't necessarily have to have anything in common. One can go mainstream like 'Basketball Eye' or obscure like 'Curler's Toe'. Try some at home. Make it a party game. Then send in your submissions and let's see if we can get them marketed. Heck, we can even start a reality show to rival 'American Idol'!

So you don't have to be a swimmer to get 'Swimmer's Ear'. You can get swimmer's ear from simply wading or doing repeated cannon balls. You can even get swimmer's ear on dry land. But getting the head immersed in water can increase the risk.

The medical term for 'swimmer's ear' is 'otitis externa'. 'Oto' means ear. '-itis' means inflammation. 'Externa' refers to the outer part. Put them all together and we have 'inflammation of the outer ear'. In this specific case, 'inflammation' almost always means infection.

The ear is like a trilogy: it has three parts. The first part is from the outside (i.e., the hole where nothing 'smaller than your elbow' is supposed to go) to the ear drum. And just like the first part of any trilogy, it is simple, straight forward, and very much an 'origin' story. In this case, it is the origin of the hearing process. (I'm just glad the first part did so well at the box office, otherwise we would not have had parts II and III and we would all be living in a silent world.)

The outer ear is really just a tube that carries sound towards the ear drum. Since it is open to the outside world, water, dust, car keys and other foreign items can find their way in. Sometimes these foreign elements cause an infection in the outer ear.

The result is redness, swelling, and pain. In some cases, goop starts to come out of the ear. ('Goop' is a medical term for anything liquid that oozes from an infected orifice.)

Since the infection is restricted to the outer part of the ear, it is accessible from the outside. Antibiotic drops can take the treatment directly to the source and start killing the bugs.

Keeping water and other foreign items from getting into the outer ear can help prevent swimmer's ear. Wearing ear plugs when in water works well. There are also special drops that can help 'dry' out the ear canal after exposure to water. These can be helpful, too.

So we see that swimmer's ear is an equal-opportunity infection. It does not discriminate on the basis of athletic ability, occupation, political affiliation, or social status. I suppose we could all learn something from that. I just wish it used its powers for good instead of evil.

An Awkward Situation

2014 A.D. Still no floating cars but my daughter's turning nine and she is due to go in for her well-child—excuse me—her well 'princess' check. One of the things that's going to happen is that she'll get her first of a three series vaccine aimed at preventing cervical cancer. This vaccine has been out since late 2006, and for the last nine years I've been rehearsing in my mind how to approach this situation when the time comes. And here we are.

I figure she's old enough to be more involved and informed about her healthcare so I rehearsed the following speech:

> 'So we're going to go see the doctor to make sure you're growing normally and to do what we can to keep you from getting sick. Most likely you'll need to get a shot to keep you from getting sick. When girls get older—like 35—some of them choose to have sex with boys—well, hopefully they'll be grown, emotionally mature men by that time but that's no guarantee. Anyway, sometimes women can get sick and even get cancer from having sex with men and this shot can help prevent that. Do you understand? That's my girl.'

But most likely it'll go something like this:

- So we're going to the doctor's today for your visit.
- Will I get a shot?
- (shift from foot to foot. Choke back a tear. Mumble) Yes.
- It's OK, daddy. I'm sure you won't cry this time.
- Will I get a toy?
- No, Daddy. The toys are only for kids. But maybe you can have a sticker.
    So why am I getting a shot?

- Well, it's because—er—so you won't get sick.
- Like a cold?
- (seizing the opportunity) Oh no. We don't have a vaccine for the common cold. You see, the common cold is caused by hundreds, if not thousands, of different viruses that mutate continually. This makes it nearly impossible—
- What are we having for dinner?
- (Saved!) I don't know, what are you in the mood for?

As mentioned in 'Thank You, Dr. P' (see chapter herein), cervical cancer is caused by a virus that women get from having sex with men. It's called the Human Papilloma Virus, HPV for short. This is also the same virus that causes warts. There are hundreds of 'strains', meaning kinds, of HPV. Fortunately, only a handful can cause cancer and of that handful, four types in particular are the most common cause of cervical cancer.

There is a new vaccine that can protect women from this virus, specifically the four kinds most likely to cause cervical cancer. It's approved for girls/women 9-26 years of age. The idea is to vaccinate girls before they become sexually active in order to prevent the disease.

The vaccine is a series of three injections: After the first vaccine, the second one is given in one month and the third is given in six months.

Depending on the child, some discussion might need to take place regarding the reasons for the vaccine. It might be an uncomfortable conversation, but it can also be a good opportunity to open discussion on an important topic.

For the parents of boys out there, don't breathe too easily yet. The vaccine is currently being researched for use in boys and I suspect that soon enough parents of boys will be facing a similarly awkward situation.

Some groups have expressed concern that the vaccine will encourage promiscuity among teenagers and young adults. Similar concerns have been expressed in the past—and continue to be expressed—about sex education and access to birth control. But when research has been done to investigate the impact of sex education and access to birth control on how soon people have intercourse, there was no effect. People with access to birth control and sex education didn't start having sex any sooner than people who weren't exposed to that information. It seems that the decision of whether or when to have sex is more complicated than simply avoiding pregnancy or disease.

AYSO—'Tis the Season

Abundant summer sun and timed sprinklers bring about a wondrous transformation to local parks, schools and greenbelts. By 'greenbelt' I don't mean the long strip of fabric you get to tie around your waste after breaking a board with your foot as an orange belt. 'Greenbelt' is a term I have just recently become familiar with. As I put in my request for practice space for the American Youth Soccer Organization (AYSO) team I coach, one of my options is to choose a 'greenbelt'. Apparently, all those random patches of grass that are not officially parks, i.e., they don't have a brown wooden sign with a name on it, would be considered greenbelts. Although in our coastal desert, at this time of year, they look more like brown belts. And by 'brown belt' I don't mean someone who is one level below a black belt.

But I digress.

Yes, I feel magic in the air this time of year—beyond the beaming faces of parents whose children have just resumed school. It's AYSO season and every park, school, and 'greenbelt' is covered with children of all ages in colorful neon outfits kicking a ball around.

This is the one time of year when soccer is truly on the forefront of American consciousness, even more than during the FIFA World Cup. (Why, Zidane? Why?!)

Kids lie awake in bed late on a Friday night, filled with excitement and anticipation of what they will have for their half-time snack the next day. Parents stay awake late on Fridays wondering what they're going to bring for half-time snack the next day. Coaches lie awake going over line-ups and strategies and praying to the gods of all major religions (and some minor ones) for a good outcome. Referees lie awake reviewing in their minds the self-defense moves they learned in referee class.

Besides sleepless Friday nights, half-time snacks, and nervous coaches and referees, AYSO season can also brings with it injuries.

Fortunately, children are limber enough that they don't tend to get sprains, strains and pulled muscles like adults do. They can, however, get 'overuse' injuries. An 'overuse' injury, as the name suggests, is not caused by a specific event, such as getting hit or twisting a joint, but it occurs from doing the same activity over and over again.

One such injury is Sever's disease which has nothing to do with removing body parts. It's named, I assume, after Dr. Sever who first discovered it. What a great name that is for a surgeon. (Other great medical names: Dr. Payne—anesthesia, Dr. Gross—pathology, and Dr. Brown—gastroenterology.)

Sever's disease is inflammation of the Achilles tendon where it inserts into the back of the heel. The Achilles tendon is the rope-like structure just below the calf muscle. It's also where the Greek Mythological hero Achilles got hit with an arrow. The arrow, tragically, brought about the hero's demise. After that, the streets of Athens were filled with anti-bow-and-arrow demonstrations and I believe it cost the congressman the election that year.

Children have a growth plate on the back of their heel and it can get irritated with repeated activity. A 'growth plate', as the name implies, is the part of the bone that allows the bone to grow longer. Children with Sever's disease have pain in their heels that gets worse with activity.

The treatment for Sever's disease (and any other overuse injury for that matter) is rest, ice, and anti-inflammatories. Relative rest also works, i.e., doing the same activity, but on a less intense scale. Ibuprofen works well to reduce the inflammation. Applying ice after practices and games is also helpful. Sever's disease can take up to six weeks to resolve.

So good luck to everyone every weekend. Hope to see you on the field and here's wishing us all a safe and injury-free soccer season. Let the good times roll towards the other team's goal just beyond the reach of their goalkeeper.

Baby Blues, Reds, and Purples

Clouds move in. The sky grows dark and a distant rumble is heard. The storm is coming. I feel it in my bones like a dog anticipating an earthquake. His face grimaces; the legs bend. He inhales. I grab onto a doorframe for dear life as the wail hits me with gale force winds of up to 150 miles per hour.

Fighting the wind, I stammer to the child, pick him up and start my repertoire of comfort measures. Put him on the shoulder. Rock him. Walk and rock. Walk, rock and sing. Walk, rock and sing while bouncing. Hold him like a football while doing the graveyard dance from Thriller (being ever vigilant not to slam the ball at the end). Meanwhile, he is turning all the colors of the rainbow and goes for what seems like minutes in between howls.

Normally, I would panic. And many are the times that I did when my now-two-year-old daughter threw her fits at the tender age of four weeks. I would undress her completely, searching frantically for a strangled appendage. Finding all parts present and pink was almost disappointing. What was going on? Where was the hot metal poker that was jabbing her?

Then the medical part of my brain would kick in, coolly analyzing that the likelihood of something being seriously wrong is very slim. Why, she was just smiling and eating ten minutes ago! She showed no signs of illness. She was a happy, thriving newborn and now she's possessed. The visceral, new-parent part of my brain would curse for not having picked up holy water on the way home. Surely the church wouldn't open its doors at 2 a.m. Or would they? It *is* an emergency.

But now I'm a seasoned veteran (with the emotional and psychological scars to prove it). I know the storm will pass. And sure enough, a toot and a burp later, the sky clears, the sun comes out and the birds start chirping 'Morning Has Broken' in three-part harmony.

So why do newborns put their parents through such ordeals? One theory is that it has to do with their intestines. It seems reasonable since the episodes are relieved by expulsion of gas and cheese curds.

A good friend told me that since humans walk upright and the pelvis had to be tilted to accommodate, human babies are born two months premature. As a result, the intestines aren't developed enough and have trouble digesting. This seems logical considering that the howling storms magically stop at two months.

My theory is that this is a test put on by Mother Nature: If all members of the family are still alive and in one piece after two months, then you are worthy of the baby.

Treatment regimens for these newborn bouts of fury are as varied as the parents who suffer through them. Various medications, teas, sugar drinks, etc., have been used through the years. Simethicone (Mylicon) can (theoretically) break up bigger gas bubbles into smaller ones and relieve symptoms. In my own personal experience, it has definitely given me something to do while I wait for the baby to calm down.

The important thing to keep in mind is to avoid liquids with caffeine and to limit any non-breast milk/formula fluids to less than two ounces a day. Any more fluid can wash the salts out of a baby's blood, causing them to become gravely ill.

So a word of encouragement and hope to new parents, and a word of caution to parents to be: Beware the storms! They will come. But just as sure as they come, they will pass. If the child was perfectly happy and feeding well ten minutes prior to the demonic transformation, chances are there is nothing seriously wrong with the child and it's simply a matter of time before the demons exorcise themselves.

(<u>Author's Note</u>: These newborn episodes of fury are very different than 'colic' which is an entirely different meteorological phenomenon. But that is a topic for a different day.)

The Beast Within

Like a giant prehistoric worm or a creature out of a sci-fi movie (like the one that swallowed the Millennium Falcon in Episode V), the colon writhes and undulates in the abdomen, sucking fluid out of intestinal products and preparing it for export.

Unlike some other body organs, the colon truly has a mind of its own. It's called the 'enteric nervous system'. Calling it a 'mind' is actually being very generous. It's more like a collection of nerves that work together in a coordinated manner—like an automatic sausage maker. It's a very ancient system as befits a pre-historic worm.

One of my medical school attendings once described the colon as an organ of convenience. It's simply a storage/fluid recycling place for intestinal stuffing until the appropriate time at which it can be expelled. One could easily live without the colon, provided one drank some extra fluid and had a container in which to put the constant stream of intestinal waste. But I would never say that directly to a colon. In fact, I hope I never have to say *anything* directly to a colon.

The colon, like so many other ancient beings, can get lazy sometimes. When it does, we experience constipation. Constipation takes many forms: some people experience it as having hard stools. Some feel like they haven't gotten everything out, and some have to strain. Frequency is not a part of it. Normal colons can export three times a day to every three days.

So what can one do when the beast within decides to take a holiday? A trip to the local drug store will reveal a dizzying array of options. They tend to fall into three general categories: fiber, stool softeners, and laxatives.

Fiber is the same stuff that's in fruits, vegetables, 'whole grains', and corrugated cardboard. It's the part of these foods that is not digested. The colon is excited when it gets to play with fiber. It loves it and squeezes it and pets it and calls it 'George'. Then it sends it out into the real world with a tearful good-bye.

Stool softeners are like the colonic version of a Slip and Slide. For those of you who didn't watch commercials during He-Man, the Slip and Slide is a rectangular tarp that has tubes running down either side of it. When connected to a garden hose, the tubing sprays water onto the tarp. Then, the beaming, happy, lean kids in the commercial would take turns (very politely) running and gliding on their bellies all the way down the tarp. I believe the straight-toothed muscular dad and the curvaceous mother with ivory skin would take turns as well. Oh, how I wish I lived in that neighborhood!

So stool softeners make things slippery inside the colon. The colon tries to hold on to stool-softened waste, but it keeps slipping through its grips like a fish through the hands of a cartoon character. And the next thing you know, the fish is gone.

Then there are the laxatives. These are the colonic equivalent of a triple no-foam-hazelnut-whip-soy-non-fat latte. It gets the colon peristalting in spite of itself. The laxatives work well, but just like the triple no-foam-hazelnut-whip-soy-non-fat latte, too much can actually cause harm. Laxatives, if used regularly, can damage the inside of the colon.

So if the beast within decides to snooze on the job, there are many ways to get it going again—some gentle, and some not so gentle. But like any ancient animal, the colon likes a routine. Keeping evacuation times regular can help keep the colon regular and purring like a contented cat. And just like with cats, the distinction between master and beast can be very gray indeed.

The Beast Within Gets Irate

One good thing about writing a bi-monthly column for a newspaper is that I get to use the word 'fortnight'. I used to think that 'fortnight' meant forty nights (as in Moses roamed the desert for a fortnight), but now I know it means two weeks (i.e., fourteen nights). For the sake of clarity, I say we change the spelling to 'fourt'night'. That way, we free up 'fortnight' for all those occasions when we need a quick expression for forty nights.

Given the theme of this chapter's topic, we could have ourselves a colonic 'fortnight'. If our fortnight also involved dramatic cleansing by way of a forceful introduction of large volumes of fluid, then we'd have a 'high colonic fortnight'.

But I digress.

When the beast within gets lazy, we experience constipation (see previous chapter). But sometimes the beast within starts to behave like a really stressed out, emotionally unstable regional manager. The pressure from the supervisor above (the brain) and the employees below (ingested foods) really starts to get to it and it starts to behave erratically. Sometimes it's nice and calm, sometimes it's overly laid back, and sometimes it gets frantic like a chipmunk in detox.

As hosts of this erratic entity, we experience periods of constipation, alternated by diarrhea. There's usually a lot of 'gassiness' and cramping involved. These are typically triggered by eating and stress.

What do we call this constellation of symptoms brought about by an irritated bowel? How about 'Irritable Bowel Syndrome' or 'IBS' for short. It's simple, straight-forward and can be used as a free-standing sentence.

Like any overly stressed, emotionally unstable regional manager, the colon will deny that anything's wrong. All tests, scopes, biopsies and cultures of an irritated colon come back normal.

The syndrome is caused by the colon (and bowels) spasming and contracting in an uncoordinated manner. A normal colon moves like an earth worm. All the muscles along it contract in a coordinated manner to move it forward. An irritable bowel moves like an earthworm that has had too much to drink. The muscles contract, but out of order, and the worm goes nowhere. Eventually, a worm cop pulls it over and asks if it has been drinking which the worm invariably denies. 'No ociffer. I haven't drink binking.' The worm ends up spending the night in a drunk tank with a couple of moths dressed up as monarch butterflies who try to proposition it.

So people with IBS feel gassy, bloated, and crampy. They have constipation and, at times, diarrhea.

This is very different from Inflammatory Bowel Disease (IBD) which is actual inflammation of the bowel. The colon in IBD usually bleeds and blood tests and endoscopies confirm inflammation.

The treatments for IBS are as varied as the colons that have it. The most significant factor is stress control. Since the colon has a mind of its own, it's very sensitive to its surroundings. So if the person as a whole is stressed out, the colon will be stressed out, too.

Certain foods can worsen IBS. Fiber supplements, specifically psyllium, can be helpful. Psyllium can soften hard stools and harden soft stools. It's very smart for a fiber supplement.

As uncomfortable as IBS may be, it is not a harmful condition. It does not increase one's risk of any serious colon or health problems in the future.

So when the beast within starts to get irate, the best bet is to stay calm. Ask it to talk about its feelings, keeping in mind that we are dealing with an organism that has a very primitive way of communicating. Perhaps this can be carried out in the form of a culinary Q&A. Insert a food item through the mouth and wait to see what the colon has to say about it; then write down the response. This can help determine if there are any particular foods to which the colon takes exception. Also, keeping the corporate 'head' off its back can help.

The angry outbursts and emotional liability will still happen, but probably not as often and not as intensely—which is fine, considering that if we were to fire this regional manager, we'd have a heck of a time finding a replacement.

Bee Owies

(_Author's Note_: *During my World Cup-induced soccer incapacitation, I asked my four-and-a-half-year-old daughter to write my column for me. A word to the wise: a four-and-half-year-old's writing needs a lot of editing.*

Daddy's watching soccer. He told me to write his words. He said he writes words about owies. I want to write words about owies, too. Bees give you owies. You have to be careful and only look with your eyes. No touch.

When I get an owie from a bee, I don't cry 'cause I'm a big girl. My brother cries but that's OK 'cause he's a little baby and he doesn't want to play with my kitty 'cause it's *my* kitty and he has a doggie, but I'm nice and I share.

Bees sting you with their butt. Heheheh I said butt. Heheheh. Did you say butt? Heheheh. I didn't say—*[edited to preserve article length.]*

You have to get mommy or daddy to help you get the stinger out. That's what it's called—a stinger. And you don't squeeze it 'cause that gives you more owies. Daddy uses his nail to take it out.

[She means 'scratch' it out.]

Or you can use daddy's small grabby tool *[tweezers]* to pull it out.

[More specifically, the bee's stinger looks like a comma. The upper, round part, is the poison sac. Grab the bottom part with the tweezers to remove.]

You take the stinger and put it in the trash veeerrry carefully like this.

[She's walking on her tip-toes and placing an imaginary crumpled tissue in an imaginary trash can.]

So the man comes and takes it in the garbage truck and my little brother runs outside to say hi to the garbage truck.

But the owie gets red and big. And then mommy and daddy give you special owie medicine in the baby cup and another owie medicine in a baby cup and that makes it all better.

[She means ibuprofen (Advil, Motrin) for inflammation and pain, and diphenhydramine (Benadryl) for the allergic reaction that causes part of the swelling and redness. Diphenhydramine should be taken mainly at night because of the sedating effects. Loratadine (Claritin) can be taken during the day as an anti-histamine since it is non-sedating.]

Daddy, it's my turn now! I do it! You go watch soccer. Sometimes when the bee stings you, you get an owie in your throat and that's very bad 'cause when you have an owie in your throat, then Tinkerbell goes down, down, down to the fairies in the park.

[What she's trying to say is that some people have allergic reactions to bee stings which winds up causing swelling in the throat and difficulty breathing. This is very different from a 'local' reaction, aka redness and swelling, at the site of the sting which everyone gets.]

Daddy, you listen to my words! It's my turn! You go away!.

[But this is a very important point. No matter how red or swollen the bee sting site is, it's still considered a 'local reaction'. This is very different from a systemic, aka 'allergic', reaction where the effect of the bee sting is felt in a different location (i.e., the throat) than where the stinger entered the body. An 'allergic' reaction.]

Meow. Meeeooooowww.

[She's pretending to be a kitty.]

The kitty's name is Kertchel.

[The point still needs to be made that an allergic reaction is a medical emergency and needs to be treated right away.]

Now I'm going to watch Curious George.

[No, she's not. There's twenty minutes left in the game.]

I want to watch Curious George!

[But it's tied and anything could happen!.]

I want to watch CURIOUS GEORGE!!

[Sigh. I hope they show a rerun.]

Beware of Billboards on the Information Superhighway

What was life like before the internet? I picture grainy footage in sepia of dirt roads and horse-drawn carriages. Did people really look up numbers in phone books? Did people really go to travel agents to find good deals on airfare? Did people (present company excluded) really go to a store to partake in the skin trade? And I'm not talking about fur coats or derm abrasion—if you catch my drift.

For some people, the internet has become such an integral part of their lives that the worst part about spending a week in the Himalayas would be having to use dial-up. The internet is also many people's first choice for getting health information. It is certainly more convenient and less intimidating than trying to get a hold of a doctor. But while the internet has increased the volume of information, it hasn't done much about its accuracy. The anonymity of the web makes it difficult to hold parties accountable for the information put forth.

There is such a wealth of information on the web that it's difficult to know where to begin. Most commonly, people use 'search engines' like Google or Yahoo, type in a word, and check the results. For example, they would type 'headache' under Google and be confronted with 83,300,000 results which in and of itself is enough to give someone a headache. Ironically, one of the sites could be *www.websearchescauseheadaches.com*.

Another issue is that the information on the web lacks perspective. Rare diseases get just as much cyberspace time as very common ones. For example, fatigue is much more likely to be caused by depression than African Sleeping Sickness. Yet, the search engine doesn't necessarily discriminate based on prevalence. And since most people (present company included) tend to assume the worst, it can send people into a panic over relatively harmless conditions.

It is also important to keep in mind the source of the information. If someone is looking for information on iron supplements, visiting *www.*

stepunclesagainstironsupplements.org, might give a somewhat biased view, whereas information from the American Dietetic Association might be a bit more balanced. That is not to be confused with the American Diabetic Association which has no information on iron supplements, but is loaded with information on diabetes.

Fortunately, there are some web sites that are more user-friendly for those looking for reliable health information.

The government has set up a site, *www.healthfinder.gov*, which is a link to other reputable sites. If the government's doing it, it means that we're paying for it, so we might as well use it.

The American Academy of Family Physicians has a site, *www.familydoctor. org*, which is another good resource. It contains useful information and also has links to other reputable and reliable sites.

The Center for Disease Control (CDC) web site, *www.cdc.gov*, has good information on illnesses, travel health, and vaccinations. Remember avian flu? Mad cow? The recent outbreaks of measles and whooping cough? Even though we don't hear about them in the mainstream media, the CDC continues to keep track and you can get updated information on their web site.

Another popular web site is WebMD which incidentally has nothing to do with the state of Maryland. It seems to have good, reliable information as well.

So the next time you turn to the computer for information about a health issue, consider using one of these health-specific sites rather than a general search engine. You might find the results much more relevant and easier to decipher. While you're on the web, you might as well search for cheap fares to Hawaii while looking up the phone number for a good deli—and NOTHING else (wink, wink).

Blood Profiling

Knowing one's blood type these days is like knowing that the dog that bit you was brown with pointy ears. While that does narrow the list of suspects, more descriptive characteristics are needed. People who know their blood type know the letter and the positive/negative sign. (The positive is not a connotation of certainty.) But there are many more characteristics that make up a blood type. So knowing one's blood type these days is more a matter of curiosity than medical necessity.

But why the big fuss about blood types anyway? To find the answer, one need look no further than the white blood cells. The white blood cells are the peace-keeping forces of the body. Even though they are called 'white' and may appear 'white' (—ish) under a microscope, they are microscopic plasmic clumps of destruction. They will destroy anything they find remotely suspicious.

Imagine the white blood cells as highly trained Special Forces units charged with keeping intruders out of the body. They want to leave the body's own red blood cells alone, yet rid the body of foreign red blood cells. But how can they tell who is who? All Red blood cells look like little red Frisbees. That's where the blood type comes in.

During their intense white-cell boot camp, the white blood cells are thoroughly briefed on the markings of the body's own blood type, including the letter, the positive/negative sign, and many other distinguishing markers. They do drills where they float down a simulation blood vessel and have to destroy cardboard cutouts of foreign red blood cells that pop out from the walls whilst leaving the domestic ones alone. The white blood cell with the fastest time gets its picture mounted on the 'wall of fame'.

Once they've received their licenses to kill, the white blood cells head out into the blood stream. They pull over red blood cells at random, ask them to step out of the vehicle and present some ID. They go back to their white blood cell patrol car and cross check the ID with their list of markers. If the red blood cell does not have the correct letter and/or positive/negative sign, it is destroyed on the spot. No paperwork. No red blood cell traffic school. No appeals.

If the letter and the positive/negative sign match, the white blood cell continues down the list of markers. If the match is only off by one or two minor markers, the red blood cell might get off with a warning—depending on the white blood cell's mood.

So if someone gets a blood transfusion that is not correctly matched, the white blood cells would be inundated with foreign red blood cells and would go on a destruction spree. This would start a chain reaction that could eventually end up killing the very body these white blood cells are trying to defend. (The irony is completely lost on them.) This is called a 'transfusion reaction'.

Therefore, when someone needs a transfusion, the lab tries to find as close a match to the patient's blood as possible. This screening goes way beyond the letter and the positive/negative sign of the blood type. This is why people, in general, no longer need to know their blood types to give or receive blood.

There are two exceptions, however. One is pregnant women who have already had a child. If their blood type is positive and the fetus' blood type is negative (or vice versa), that could set off a transfusion reaction and endanger the fetus' life. This is why blood typing is a routine part of the care of pregnant women.

The other is contestants on 'Survivor' who would be on a deserted island with no access to medical care. They might want to know their own (and everyone else's) blood type in case they have to give or receive blood using hypodermics made of bamboo.

As for the rest of us, we needn't worry.

Blowing Smoke

Thanks to modern DVR (Digital Video Recorder) technology, I haven't watched a commercial in years—excluding the time when I recorded the Super Bowl and fast-forwarded the game. But back in the day when we had to sit through commercials with program breaks, nothing would get me more riled up than direct-to-consumer ads for medications. I would turn red and every muscle in my body would twitch as if I were bench pressing a 35-pound bar. Study after study has shown that direct-to-consumer advertising of medications is nothing but an emotional plea devoid of any real scientific information that drives up healthcare costs.

But there was one emotional plea devoid of any real scientific information that I was actually happy about. I never saw the ad but heard about it through a few patients. These were people who smoked and wanted to quit. The medication in question was varenicline aka Chantix.

I'm all for anything that helps smokers take the next step towards quitting. If a parade of monkeys doing the chicken dance watched by chickens doing the monkey dance makes someone want to quit, I'll be the first to sign up for a monkey suit. (I don't chicken very well and I don't eat monkey.)

But varenicline is not the only option when it comes to quitting smoking—it's just the one with the biggest advertising budget. There is another prescription medication, bupropion aka Wellbutrin aka Zyban, that can help. They each have a fifty percent chance of helping someone succeed which may not sound like a lot, but when it comes to something as addictive as cigarettes, and the enormous health benefits that result from quitting smoking, fifty percent is Olympic Gold!

Besides prescription medications, there are also various forms of nicotine replacement. Nicotine replacement comes in patches, gum, lozenges, and inhalers. The patch delivers a steady, reliable stream of nicotine to the body, much like floating on an inner tube down the meandering pool of an all-inclusive resort, sipping an umbrella drink while a cabana person spritzes one with cool rose water—or so I'm told.

Nicotine gum, lozenges and inhalers are more like white water rafting on a level IV river (the IV stands for 'I'Ve gotta get me off this flimsy boat!') with peaks and valleys. They offer more episodic bursts of nicotine that mimic more closely the actual smoking experience—or so the package tells me.

Then there's the miscellaneous category: This includes hypnosis, counseling, vigorous exercise, chewing on carrot sticks, cutting each cigarette in a pack to make them shorter, delaying the timing of each cigarette, having friends fill your packs with novelty exploding cigarettes, etc.

All these options (medication, nicotine replacement and miscellany) can be mixed and matched to make finite combinations to achieve maximum effectiveness. There is no right or wrong way to do it, as long as it gets done.

To that end, I say we set up neighborhood squads. We could call them the 'Cessation Sensations'. (In the evenings, they could dress up in glittery outfits, sing Motown and not have to change their name!) During the day they would go to smokers' homes and places of work and offer them a percentage of the healthcare money they would save for every day they don't smoke. Even if we only offer them fifty percent, it would still turn out to be a huge financial incentive for the smokers and would save loads of healthcare money in the long run.

So I urge all smokers out there to give it a shot. The options are plenty and all you have to lose are years of ill health and a skinny wallet. Perhaps avoiding the 'Cessation Sensations' rendition of 'Stop! In the Name of Love' will be motivation enough.

Board Stiff

I've been studying for my Family Practice Boards for the last two weeks. (How quickly seven years have gone by!) I've set a goal of one hour a day. And oh, how it has brought back a flood of memories from medical school and residency. As soon as I sit down to study, a thousand thoughts enter my mind:

'I really should clean the living room.'
'What was the name of that movie with Tom Hanks and Meg Ryan? Not *Sleepless in Seattle*. Not *You've Got Mail*. The other one.'
'Is the stove on? I should really check. It's a fire hazard.'

Once the place is immaculately clean, the internet has told me, 'Joe Versus the Volcano', and the stove is checked, it's back to studying. That's when the music starts. Even if it's a song I like, after about the eighth time through, it starts to get old. All my mental efforts at silencing it only yield a ten-second pause, after which the song resumes exactly where I stopped it. It's like an unstoppable mental iPod.

So why would I put myself through such an ordeal when my brain is so clearly against it? It's not like I really need Board Certification to practice medicine. Before I answer that question, let's clarify what Board Certification means.

Every specialty has a Board. A Board is a governing body—of sorts. These Boards have special secret names like The American Board of Family Practice, the American Board of Orthopaedic Surgery, or the American Board of Pediatrics. What those names stand for is anyone's guess, but one thing we do know is that these Boards design and administer a test that enables a physician to become 'Board Certified'.

I like to think that the original name for these governing bodies was the Boreds because they were started by a group of physicians who had nothing better to do. The name was later changed to the Boards because that's what they used to discipline physicians who didn't pass the test. But I don't think that's true.

Once the Board has administered the test to its disciples, it corrects them and goes on to inform anyone and everyone via the internet, phone request, or sticky notes on refrigerators, which physicians have passed the test.

As mentioned before, a physician can still practice medicine without being a part of the American Board of Their Specialty. However, in reality, it's about as optional as a reservation at a local hot spot on a Saturday night. Sure, one can try to go and wait for a table, but will most likely wind up spending the night out in the cold watching various other groups/couples go in and out of the establishment. And no matter how many times one emphasizes that the name is *Doctor* Javanbakht (Board Certified Family Physician), it makes little difference.

Physicians who are not Board Certified are finding themselves standing out in the cold more and more while Board Certified Physicians get privileges at hospitals, contracts with insurance companies, and employment at big clinics.

The one thing we can say with great confidence about Board Certified Physicians is that they're great test takers. We can also say that they've had to review current practice standards for their field in order to prepare for the test. (Although there are some outstanding test takers out there who get away with little or no review. I hate them.)

So now that I have spent precious studying time completing this chapter, I shall go clean out the attic. It's been three years and I simply cannot study until it's done. First, I'll have to find out where the attic is. I just hope that at this time next year, I won't be writing an article on what it's like being a non-Board Certified Family Physician.

(*Editor's Note: Dr. Javanbakht did pass his Board Certification in Family Medicine and is now the proud owner of a sticky note on his refrigerator to remind. him. Unfortunately, he's still looking for his attic.*)

Bone-Building Buddies

After writing the chapter on vitamin D (see chapter herein), I was accosted by multiple hate emails in my inbox, numerous angry tweets on my phone, and a few brown paper bags on fire on my front door. That's what I get for messing with the Calcium Support Coalition aka CaSCo. They asked me who did I think I was, writing an article on vitamin D without giving equal time to calcium. I told them they were mighty high on themselves for an organization that is a near homonym for a discount warehouse store.

I cannot divulge in print the details of what ensued, but let's just say they made me a discount offer in bulk that I could not refuse. So this chapter is on vitamin D's Bone-Building Buddy (BBB), calcium.

Calcium and vitamin D have been close since time immemorial. Rumor has it that one of them has a half-heart necklace with 'vita-' and 'calc-' on it and the other has the other half of the heart necklace with '-min D' and '-ium' on it. Scientists have given up trying to determine who has which necklace because it doesn't really matter.

One of the main effects of vitamin D on the body is that it makes the intestines much more efficient at absorbing calcium. Calcium levels in the blood are very important in helping the body work properly. If the blood calcium level is too high, it can cause some vague symptoms like fatigue, confusion and body aches. If the blood calcium level is too low, it can cause other vague symptoms like anxiety, numbness and muscle cramps. However, having abnormal calcium levels is very rare. Many other conditions, such as parenthood, can cause the same symptoms. Nevertheless, it is in the body's best interest to keep very tight control on blood calcium levels.

To accomplish this, the body has set up an elaborate system of hormones and feedback loops to keep calcium at an appropriate level. For example, after one eats a high calcium item such as milk or yogurt, calcium levels rise in the blood. The body doesn't want to waste precious calcium and thus tries to absorb as much of it as it can. To keep blood levels of calcium from continuously rising, the body needs to have a place to put the extra calcium.

Enter the bones.

Besides being sturdy structures that muscles attach to, give our bodies rigidity, and give us facial features whose altitudes we can admire, bones are a vast reservoir of calcium. When blood levels of calcium climb after a meal, the body starts putting the extra calcium into the bones.

The other organ that helps control calcium levels is the kidney. When calcium levels rise, the kidneys start to dump out extra calcium in the urine. This is why it is difficult to overdose on calcium, although this is not to be taken as a challenge to try.

Conversely, when calcium levels start to drop, i.e., when people do not consume enough of it, the reverse process puts calcium back into the blood stream. In other words, the bones start to release calcium into the blood stream and the kidneys keep calcium from going out with the urine. So the body will draw as much calcium from bones as it needs to, even to the point of making the bones thin, to keep the blood level stable. That is why calcium intake is so important in post-menopausal women.

This is also why a calcium blood test is not a good measure of how much calcium one is eating. The body will do what it can to keep the blood level of calcium correct regardless of the amount consumed.

So as we become more conscientious about our intake of vitamin D, let's not forget it's BBB, calcium. One without the other just doesn't have the same effect. And I'd like to offer my humblest apologies to CaSCo for last fortnight's oversight. I assure them it will never happen again and I sincerely hope that my Costco card will be returned to me, unharmed.

Bone Density

Many seniors have advised me not to get old. To that end, I've had multiple portraits of me commissioned in the hopes that one of them will take over the aging duties. Of all the chronic diseases that can befall the elderly, broken hips are one of the more serious. In fact, broken hips are common and dangerous enough to warrant their own screening test: the Bone Density Study.

The bone density study is a special X-ray that determines how strong the bones are. The less strong the bones, the more likely they are to break. A typical bone density study checks the hip and the lower back.

The results classify the bone as normal (aka titanium grade), osteopenia (aka iron) and osteoporosis (aka aluminum.)

If one gets a normal result on a bone density test, one can leap for joy, resting assured that the hip will not break upon landing. But one must continue to consume calcium and vitamin D to keep the bones strong.

If the result is osteopenia, one can still leap for joy, but preferably a smaller leap on level ground. Osteopenia means that the bones are weakened, but not necessarily at higher risk of fracture. One must continue to consume calcium and vitamin D and engage in weight-bearing exercise. One must also recheck the bone density every one to two years.

If one has osteoporosis, not only must one not leap with any kind of emotion, but one must stand clear of others leaping with joy, for fear of being knocked to the ground. Osteoporosis means that one is at risk of breaking a bone if one falls. One must continue to consume calcium and vitamin D, engage in weight-bearing exercise, recheck the bone density in one to two years, and start taking medications to prevent worsening of the osteoporosis.

But osteoporosis is not an equal opportunity malady. That is why not everyone needs to get a bone density screening. Women are affected far more commonly than men; therefore, they are the ones who would need screening.

A man might need a bone density screening if he has certain risk factors, such as long-term oral steroid use, but the average man doesn't need screening.

And even among women, there are those who are at higher risk of osteoporosis. Slender women, and women of Caucasian and Asian decent, are at higher risk and should be screened more aggressively.

Screening for average-risk women starts at around 65 years of age. For higher risk women, it might be started sooner.

So consult your healthcare provider to see if bone density screening is right for you. Then, consider whether or not to leap.

Bronchitis

Attention readers: I'm about to reveal a major medical secret. Sure, I've been sworn to secrecy and the dreaded medical police could be after me, but prudence be darned! This is for the people!

The suffix—*itis*, that medical personnel toss around like it's switch grass ready to be turned into ethanol, actually means 'inflammation'. It is a wonderful suffix—as suffixes go—because it's about as committal as saying someone's 'upset'. 'Upset' could mean angry, sad, infuriated, or mildly disappointed. 'Inflammation' could mean an infection (by bacteria, virus, fungus, prions, etc.), an allergic reaction, irritation from a chemical or an attack by the body's own immune system.

Let's review some examples. Arthritis means inflammation of the arthros which is Latin for joint; sinusitis means inflammation of the sinuses; cellulitis means inflammation of the—skin. OK, so the last one was a bad example, but what about arguably the most dreaded—*itis* of all: *bronchitis*! The—*itis* that everyone tries to avoid like the plague! That most dreaded complication of common colds!

Bronchitis means inflammation of the bronchus which means small airway—not to be confused with bronchiole which means *really* small airway. Pretty clever, huh? The inflammation could be from asthma, emphysema, virus, bacteria, chemicals, smoking or fungi just to name a few. Regardless of the cause, an inflamed bronchus gets a thickened lining and starts to produce sputum aka phlegm. The color can be clear, frothy, green, red or purple—if you have a taste for grape popsicles. There is also coughing and sometimes wheezing.

Bronchitis comes in two major varieties: acute and chronic. Acute bronchitis is what most people get following a cold. This is almost always caused by a virus. Chronic bronchitis is entirely different. It's defined as having sputum for three months out of a two-year period. (Even the medical profession is obsessed with sputum!) People who smoke and some people with asthma have chronic bronchitis. To make it even more confusing, it is possible for someone with chronic bronchitis to get acute bronchitis. This is called Acute Exacerbation of Chronic Bronchitis—AECB for short. Think of it as a Christmas bonus: You still get your regular pay—or in this case, phlegm—but this is just extra on top of that.

So how does one treat bronchitis?

Acute bronchitis is easy. Like virtually all viral infections, it goes away by itself. Resting, drinking extra fluids, and using a humidifier can help. And as we all know by now, taking antibiotics for a virus is about as effective as getting a manicure to lose weight. In research, placebos work just as well as any antibiotic for acute bronchitis; so your best bet is to have a close friend or relative put a stash of sugar pills in a bottle labeled 'bronchitis medicine' and have him/her give you a seven-day course every time you come down with an episode of bronchitis. It's much cheaper than filling a prescription for antibiotics and doesn't make for resistant bacteria.

Chronic bronchitis is treated by dealing with whatever is causing the chronic bronchitis. Smokers should stop smoking. Asthmatics should take inhalers. People who are exposed to toxic fumes should wear appropriate gear or get that toaster oven cleaned once and for all.

AECB can be bacterial and may need antibiotics. If you haven't already, you'll soon start seeing advertisements 'educating' you on AECB, and encouraging you to ask your doctor to see if medication X is right for you. But heed the warnings: Side effects may include drowsiness, nausea, headache, freckles, being picked last for sports teams, missing work on Tuesdays, and singing old Frank Sinatra songs. Medication X should not be taken by pregnant or nursing women, people with crooked or overly straight teeth, or on odd days of even months. Consult your doctor if you experience unusual dreams or if people start calling you 'Morris'.

So the next time you get that cough with the phlegm, get your doctor's help in sorting out what kind of bronchitis you have. The rest is easy.

Capitation

Capitation is not what is attempted after someone is wrongly sent to the guillotine. But it is the way HMOs (Health Maintenance Organizations) do business. This is not to say that the way HMOs do business is like sending people to the guillotine. In fact, none of the major HMOs even cover guillotine treatment. If a client of theirs were to get guillotine treatment, he or she would have to pay out of pocket.

I remember the head of Pediatrics at Children's Hospital of Wisconsin (let's call him Dr. CHW) declaring to us medical students that 'capitation is evil.' I didn't quite understand what he was talking about back then, but I think I know now what he was getting at.

Here's how a 'capitated' system works: I pay my monthly HMO fees on time like the good, concerned citizen I am about losing my healthcare coverage. My HMO company keeps *some* (or a lot—depending on whom you ask) of my money and gives *some* (or a lot—depending on whom you ask) every month to my doctor, Dr. No. Under the capitated system, Dr. No gets the same amount of money each month regardless of how often I see him.

If I don't see Dr. No at all in any given month, that frees up more of his time to devise overly elaborate plans to kill off James Bond. On the other hand, if I have to go see Dr. No every day for a month, he loses a lot of money since he has less time to tend to his evil deeds which are far more lucrative than his HMO contract. (By the way, Dr. No, in spite of his dealings with murder and mayhem, is surprisingly positive with his patients; that's why I still go to him even though I can't get an appointment for three months.)

So it is to Dr. No's financial advantage to have a very large number of HMO patients who never come in. He gets his monthly check and still has all the time in the world to blackmail world leaders.

From the HMO perspective, their monthly income remains the same no matter how sick I get. It takes the 'risk' out of covering me.

I believe what Dr. CHW was concerned about was that this puts undue pressure on healthcare providers. It's no mystery that there are no business classes in medical school. (If there were, I would have likely pursued my dream of becoming a body double for Pee Wee Herman instead.) Very few doctors go into medicine because they like the business aspect of it. Yet in a capitated system, the provider must bear the burden of providing care while trying to manage the direct negative financial impact that this care will have on his/her practice.

Given this, it's understandable how most providers aren't very excited about the HMO set-up. A lot of them have simply stopped seeing HMO patients. And from what I hear, they're doing quite alright. Those who continue to take HMO patients are in a constant battle for better 'capitated' rates in order to keep their businesses solvent. (I'm referring to financial solvency and not chemicals that dissolve things. Although I'm sure the solvent industry is more solvent than medicine.)

On the plus side for patients, HMO insurance tends to have lower out-of-pocket costs compared to other types of insurance, provided that patients play by the HMO rules of seeing only who their HMO approves and only taking medications that the HMO has deemed worthy of coverage. (A process which, I hear, is modeled after the state lottery to ensure total randomness.)

So that's the dirt on capitation. It might not be pretty, but it's our reality. I just hope Dr. No continues to accept Blue Cross. Because if he doesn't, then my only remaining options would be Dr. Strangelove and Dr. Feelgood. I hear one begets the other.

Central to Obesity is
Central Obesity

The obesity epidemic continues to gather momentum. Public Health resources are strained trying to keep up. If we don't change things soon, the National Guard will have to be called in. They will block off access to high-calorie foods, check IDs and only allow those with doctor's notes down the potato chip aisle. They will stop cars randomly and force its occupants to walk. They will install secret power control devices on televisions that would automatically turn it off once it has been on for two hours a day. The Red Cross would have to set up emergency tents equipped with treadmills and racquet ball courts to accommodate the throngs of people displaced by the lack of sedentarism.

To help streamline their efforts, each National Guard officer would be deployed with a calculator. He/she would enter each person's weight in pounds, divide it by their height in inches squared, and multiply the whole thing by 703. Weight (pounds) ÷ [Height x Height (inches)] x 703 = BMI. This would help determine each person's Body Mass Index (BMI) and thus serve as a measure of their weight status. For example, a person weighing 220 lbs. who is 6 ft. 3 inches tall has a BMI of 27.5. 220 lbs. ÷ (75 x 75 inches) x 703 = 27.5.

Those with a BMI of 19-25 (and thus in the 'ideal' category) would receive all access passes. Those with a BMI of 25.1 to 29.9 (and thus in the 'overweight' category) would be tagged with GPS-enabled pedometers and monitored from a centrally located office. Those with a BMI over 30 (and thus in the 'obese' category) would be taken into special custody and would have at their disposal a team of physical therapists, nutritionists, behaviorists and maybe even some hair-stylists.

But the National Guard, with the foresight and careful planning that only comes from govern-mental institutions, would realize that the Body Mass Index has its limitations. They would also need to consider *where* somebody carries their weight.

Arnold Schwarzenegger (in his 'Terminator' days) would have most likely had a body mass index in the overweight, if not obese, range. Yet few people would dare call him overweight or obese. In fact, the Terminator came back to 'eliminate' Sarah Connor not to prevent her from having a son, but because of an unflattering comment she had made about his leather jacket.

The Terminator, as most of us recall, was very muscular. He had thighs like Grecian columns and biceps like Roman columns. His pectorals were like the stone slabs on which the Ten Commandments were written. His washboard abdomen glistened under the movie-set lights like the cobble-stoned streets of Paris after a spring shower. And all combined, I believe that if he were to eat two pounds of pure lard, that would bring his total body fat up to 1.3 pounds.

The point is that people who are very muscular weigh more and therefore have a higher BMI, but that does not mean that their health is at risk because of their weight.

In contrast, if we were to look at the Governator now (years after Terminator fame), we would find that his thighs are like the pillars of a bouncy castle, his biceps are more like water balloons, his pectorals are leaning more towards Dolly Parton's, and his abdomen would look more like an impending mudslide. This body composition might increase his health risk.

The weight that is stored in the abdominal area increases someone's risk of health complications. This is known as 'central' or 'trunkal' obesity. A simple way to measure it is to measure the smallest area around the abdomen above the belly button and below the ribs. The number for men should be less than 40 inches, and for women it should be less than 35 inches.

This measurement, along with the BMI, can help determine who is truly at risk and thus would not unjustly deny the Terminator his cherished bag of Hot Cheetos. And I think it's to everyone's benefit to keep the Terminator happy. The Governator on the other hand . . .

Chill Out On Fever

It's like that Whack-the-Gopher game at the local fair. You stand there, waiting for the little plastic rodents to raise their head so you can whack them on the head with the overly padded gopher-basher. Then when you're nice and smelly, you win a tiny stuffed animal for your date who never really liked you anyway, but just came out because she wanted to be near your friend who's double-dating with you with that girl you don't like who always seems to hang around. Isn't that always the case? But enough about my high school years.

The Whack-the-Gopher game is some people's approach to treating fevers. They stalk it, checking every two hours. As soon as it shows any sign of rearing its ugly head, they hit it with their favorite fever-reducing tool. Some like medications. Some like cooling measures, such as cool towels or showers. Some burn incense while doing the chicken dance to chase away the evil spirits. I think leaching has pretty much fallen out of favor.

Fever has been around for millions of years and we have come to see it as the enemy. Frankly, I'm not surprised. Fever takes away our appetite and makes us lie around moping on the couch—so it must be bad. (Pondering point: Where did people mope before couches were invented? I can't see it being carried out effectively on any other surface. I bet, historically, moping emerged only after the couch was invented. But I digress.)

But I'm here to play the devil's advocate (which has very high worker's comp premiums, by the way). Perhaps fever is misunderstood. What if fever is like the younger brother who starts cleaning up the cookie jar his older sister broke only to have his parents walk in and accuse him of the crime? He was really only trying to help! What if fever actually has a purpose and gives us an advantage?

As it turns out, our immune system works faster when the temperature is higher. Our white blood cells become faster killers and move more quickly when our body temperature is elevated. Also, lying around helps to conserve the energy we need to fight the infection so fever takes away our desire to move around. Certainly if you're ill, you shouldn't be wandering the forest looking for food, so our friend, fever, takes away our appetite as well.

When we get an infection, the thermostat in our brain gets reset to a higher temperature. People experience this as 'the chills'. It might seem paradoxical, but if your normal temperature is 98.6 degrees (which it isn't—a temperature of 98.6 degrees is like having 2.4 kids: Everybody has it, but nobody really has it) and all of a sudden your body wants the temperature to be at 102 degrees, your body needs to generate heat fast. So you feel cold, wrap yourself in blankets, drink hot drinks, and if that's not working—as a last resort—your body starts to twitch your muscles to generate heat. When a fever 'breaks', the brain thermostat is set back down to 98.6 degrees. Then, people feel hot and they sweat in order to bring their temperature back down.

Imagine your body as a house: Your cute little devil of a niece/nephew is visiting and, as always, he/she cranks the thermostat to 99 degrees. Next thing you know, nomads on camel-back come riding across your living room. When the camels start eating your much-treasured archived volumes of *National Geographic,* it becomes imperative to cool things down. One approach would be to open the doors and windows. This is like bathing or putting cool cloths on someone with a fever. Sure the temperature comes down, but you haven't addressed the fundamental issue: the thermostat is still set at 99. And now the furnace is mad because it has to work overtime which is clearly against its Union's rules and regs. The other approach would be to turn the thermostat down. That's what medication like acetaminophen (Tylenol) and ibuprofen (Advil, Motrin) do. A much less traumatic intervention.

So the next time you or a loved one has a fever, think twice about reaching for the faucet or the medicine cabinet. If you/they are not uncomfortable, letting the fever be is not a bad thing. It just might be the best thing you could do for them.

Chocolate and Over-the-Counter Cold Remedies

This title reminds me of those fliers in college where at the top of the page, in bold letters, was the word 'sex'. I'd eagerly run up to read them only to find out it was someone trying to sell a bicycle. But there is more to this title than mere eye-grabbing gimmickry for the chocolate enthusiast.

A few years back, I read a book entitled 'The Emperors of Chocolate' by Joel Glenn Brenner (a must-read for anyone remotely interested in chocolate, business, the business of chocolate, or the chocolate of business). In it, the author makes a very interesting point: There are a handful of components that are used to make the vast majority of chocolate bars. They are chocolate, nougat, caramel, peanut butter, and nuts. Mars Bar, Milky Way, Payday, Three Musketeers, Reece's, and Rollo, to name a few, are all made using some combination of these five components. Since there are only so many ways to combine these components (I'm sure some math enthusiast out there could give us a formula for figuring it out), candy makers search for new ways to resell the same ingredients by using various packaging and marketing techniques.

The same can be said of over-the-counter cold remedies. There are only a few ingredients that make up most over-the-counter remedies. And pharmaceutical companies are constantly looking for new ways to mix and sell these drugs.

These ingredients are: an antihistamine like diphenhydramine (Benadryl) to treat runny noses, a decongestant like phenylephrine (Neo-Synephrine) to open up stuffy noses, a medicine for pains and fever like acetaminophen (Tylenol) or ibuprofen (Advil, Motrin), and a cough medication like guaifenessin (Robitussin). For example, Contac is acetaminophen and a decongestant so it should take away pain and open up a stuffy nose. Drixoral is an antihistamine and a decongestant which should treat a runny nose and relieve stuffiness. Try the rest on your own: Theraflu is a cough suppressant, decongestant and an antihistamine, and Nyquil is acetaminophen, an antihistamine and a cough suppressant.

These ingredients have been around for a long time and are all generic and thus exceedingly inexpensive to buy. A drug company can take a few of them, mix them together, give it a fancy name, follow it with an advertising blitz and watch the profits soar!

You can make your own: Write the above ingredients on separate pieces of paper and put them in a hat. Then pull out two to three papers, go to the store, and buy a large bottle of each ingredient. The next step is to come up with a name. It's helpful to use the words 'cold', 'cough', 'sinus', or 'flu' and some type of strong prefix or suffix, like 'Neo-Sinuflu' or 'Coughin'-Ex'. Consider doubling the dose and calling it 'extra strength'. Make sure anybody looking at the packaging can tell that it's 'NEW!'

For those not interested in launching their own line of over-the-counter cold remedies but are simply looking for relief from cold and flu symptoms, consider buying the separate ingredients of your favorite cold and flu remedy instead of the fancy-labeled brand name. (They're listed in the section entitled 'ingredients' on the box/bottle.) Copy the names and look for the same stuff on the generic medicine shelf or ask the friendly pharmacy staff for assistance.

The other option is to simply get medication for specific symptoms. Try using the following table as a guide:

Symptom	**Treatment**
Stuffy nose	decongestant
Runny nose	antihistamine
Aches and pains	ibuprofen or acetaminophen
Fever	ibuprofen or acetaminophen
Cough	guaifenessin

So here's wishing everyone a happy, healthy cold and flu season. If the cold and flu should find you, feel empowered that we have medications to help the symptoms. They certainly won't cure it, but they should relieve some of the suffering.

Cholesterol: The Good, the Bad, and the Total

It was a simpler time: shoulder pads, parachute pants, John Hughes movies, girls with big bangs, boys with their underwear inside their pants and cholesterol. Just plain cholesterol—one number that directly correlated with a person's risk for heart disease. It was so simple.

Then those darned scientists had to meddle with it. (They're never satisfied, those scientific types.) They wanted to find out more about cholesterol. They took it, tweaked it, heated it, cooled it, and ran it through all kinds of machines until they found out what it was really made of.

Under the duress of scientific scrutiny, total cholesterol flung itself open to reveal its innards like that guy in *Men In Black* who had the tiny alien thingy operating in his head. When the scientists peered inside total cholesterol they saw LDL, HDL, and VLDL. But were they satisfied? Nooo. They had to take the poor defenseless components of cholesterol and start tinkering with them, too.

Much to its credit, LDL aka Low Density Lipoprotein, alias 'bad cholesterol', put up a brave fight. He kept repeating his name and serial number. But finally, he broke down and revealed his evil plans. (His alias should have been a dead giveaway.) He was intent on clogging arteries! His goal was to increase people's risk of heart disease! And he would have gotten away with it, too, if it weren't for these pesky scientists.

Next on the grill was HDL aka High Density Lipoprotein. Code name: 'good cholesterol'. He proved to be quite cooperative—too cooperative, in fact. The scientists were naturally extra suspicious of an entity that called itself 'good cholesterol' and was overly cooperative. What was his real mission? Why were his eyes so shifty? As it turned out, HDL was exceedingly honest. All his stories and alibis checked out. He was, indeed, on a mission to counter the evil LDL and help keep arteries open. He was released with a formal apology and pardon.

VLDL aka 'Very Low Density Lipoprotein', alias 'the enigma', proved to be a more difficult nut to crack. He pretended he didn't speak English. He mumbled his words and answered questions with questions. He refused to speak unless his lawyer was present. The scientists already had captured the good and bad cholesterol. What else was there? So finally they were forced to let him go. But they instructed him not to leave the area and they tapped his cell phone in case he made any international calls.

Satisfied with a job well done, the scientists were about to call it a day. But as they looked over their work station, they noticed something: Triglyceride. Like the extra piece left over after assembling a crib, triglyceride sat in the test tube feigning importance. Triglyceride, eager to distance himself from the cholesterols, was quick to volunteer information. He kept repeating that he wasn't cholesterol at all. He was something entirely different—a certain kind of fat, if you will. He was hoping to get away scot-free, but the scientists, out of spite as much as curiosity, decided to give him the full rundown. Triglyceride got the gamut: good scientist/bad scientist, sleep deprivation, and watching re-runs of *Saved by the Bell*. The scientists' persistence paid off. It turned out that triglyceride was also on a mission of clogging those arteries! And LDL yelling across the room, 'He's with me! Cloggers unite!' didn't exactly help triglyceride's cause.

So now when we get lab results, there are four numbers to review: total cholesterol, LDL, HDL, and triglycerides. A perfect reading would have a very low LDL, sky high HDL, low triglycerides and VLDL in the normal range just so we wouldn't have to deal with it. Total cholesterol used to be the hype but now has taken a back seat to its components. Alas, the world is more complex now, and no one wears parachute pants—in public. Although, I have kept mine just in case. After all, disco made a comeback.

Clarifamography

Timing is everything. In the heat of the debate over healthcare reform, while accusations of rationing healthcare were being launched back and forth like arrows in a gladiatorial battle scene, the United States Preventative Services Task Force (USPSTF) came out with its new recommendations for breast cancer screening in women. In it, they recommended against routine mammograms for women between the ages of 40-49.

Given that the USPSTF has some loose ties to the government, some people felt this was an attempt by the government to restrict women's access to mammograms and thereby reduce cost. The day the announcement was made, one could hear the collective smack of pro-health reform hands on foreheads. To them it must have been like having snow in the Bahamas during a global-warming conference.

The opponents of the current healthcare reform proposals must have been paralyzed momentarily in disbelief, which would have dissipated into suspicion. To them, it must have been like the day Jane Roe of *Roe v. Wade* turned pro-life.

In reality, the new recommendations by the USPSTF were not intended to restrict women's access to mammograms nor reduce cost.

If they could do it all again, I certainly hope the USPSTF would choose their words more carefully. The message they should have conveyed was that, after reviewing the research, they felt that *routine* (emphasis on *routine*) mammograms in women between the ages of 40-49 have a lot of false positives. This could lead to unnecessary procedures that may not increase a woman's life expectancy, not to mention the anxiety it will bring.

This is not to say that women who have risk factors—a family history of breast cancer or abnormalities on clinical breast exams—should not get mammograms. Nor does it mean that women should be barred from getting routine mammograms if they so choose.

The USPSTF is an independent panel of doctors and scientists who review the effectiveness of screening tests. It has no power to dictate how doctors and patients go about their healthcare. Many other agencies, such as the American Cancer Society (ACS), have their own recommendations for various screenings. The ACS has kept its breast cancer screening recommendations unchanged after reviewing some of the same research that the USPSTF reviewed.

So the USPSTF, the ACS, and other agencies only make recommendations. They're like the experts who advise people how to do well in a job interview. Some recommend asking meaningful questions at the end of the interview. Some recommend asking questions during the interview, when appropriate. Others recommend adding question intonations to regular sentences. Ultimately, the decision on when to ask which questions lies with the interviewee. Similarly, how often mammograms are done and at what age will ultimately be decided by patients and their doctors.

The USPSTF takes many things into consideration when making recommendations on screening procedures: evidence of effectiveness, rate of false positives, effect on life expectancy, and risks of the procedure itself, to name a few. The cost of the test is as important as its number of consonant clusters: i.e., not at all.

A female member of the panel later stated that the purpose of making the new recommendations was to clarify the strength and weaknesses of routine mammograms in women 40-49 years of age. The results were supposed to have been a more empowered patient who could make a better decision by being better informed. Instead, they may have gotten angry and confused patients who will ask for two mammograms a year just to spite them.

What effect the new recommendations will ultimately have on women's breast cancer screening remains to be seen. For now, it seems like most women and providers will carry on with annual mammograms as usual. But the one thing we have all learned from this experience is that the USPSTF needs a spokesperson. Someone who can deliver a message clearly and concisely. Without fragments. Someone who can anticipate misconceptions and clarify them before they are misconceived. They don't necessarily need a scientist or someone knowledgeable. To them, I humbly offer my services.

Cold Only *Makes* Cold

The most pleasant part of my medical education during the cold Milwaukee winters, September through June, was sitting in front of the TV on Thursday nights and watching *ER*. This is a habit I've carried to this day and still, in spite of my best efforts, I learn something new on an almost weekly basis. (*Note to self*: Send NBC bill for blatant plug.)

One particular episode had a great line. A parent was explaining her child's lung infection as being caused by being outdoors with wet hair. To this, the nurse replies, 'The only thing wet hair gives you is split ends'. I couldn't have said it better myself. In fact, I haven't.

The notion that cold air gives colds has its roots in medical history. There was a time when doctors believed colds and pneumonia came from being exposed to cold weather. That theory went out the window with the discovery of germs.

Colds are carried by viruses. Viruses are transmitted from infected individuals to non-infected individuals either through 'infectious droplets', which is fancy medical talk for the fluid that rips a hole in the tissue and smears your hand when you sneeze, or 'fomites'. A fomite is any non-living thing that can hold germs. Doorknobs and table tops are prime examples. When someone with a cold coughs into his or her hand and then touches a door knob, the cold virus sticks to the doorknob. The next person to touch the doorknob will get the virus on their hands which, in turn, will get into their body when they touch their face.

Try this experiment: the next time you're with someone, note for five minutes how many times they touch their face. It's impressive. That is why colds spread like they do. The virus is hardy and will lie on fomites waiting for its next victim. That's why hand washing is the best way to prevent catching a cold. Yes, it's even better than garlic!

So spare yourself the bad breath, get your hair wet, and go for a jog on the beach at midnight. Chill yourself to the bone. It'll only make you cold. And if you wind up *catching* a cold, it's because you had to twist the doorknob to get outside.

Consumer-Driven Healthcare

In the beginning, there was darkness. Then some other things happened and it all culminated in the creation of man. That winter, man became ill. So he went to another man for help. That other man drilled a hole in the sick man's head to release the evil spirits and thus, healthcare was born!

The man with the hole in his head gave the other man a goat and a rhubarb pie. Thus was born healthcare economics!

As any good economist (and even some bad ones) will tell you, economics is all about resources. In the goat-and-rhubarb-pie days, the patient allocated healthcare resources. That's just a fancy way of saying that patients paid for everything. Those who had goat and rhubarb pie got holes in their heads. Those who didn't have goat and rhubarb pie had to drill holes in their own heads or simply learn to live with the evil spirits.

As healthcare became more expensive, it became more and more difficult for patients to afford all the healthcare services they needed, and thus, insurance companies were born. And we all know how the managed care thing worked out!

The new buzz on Main Street these days regarding controlling healthcare costs is 'Consumer-Driven Healthcare'. Say good-bye to formulary restrictions. Say good-bye to authorizations for certain treatments, and say hello to the smorgasbord that is American healthcare.

Getting healthcare will be just like buying a pair of pants: There are no restrictions on what kind of pants anyone can buy. (Although I'm sure there are those who wish there were!) Anybody can step into Nordstrom's and buy a pair of top-of-the-line Calvin Klein slick silk slacks (try saying that ten times fast). What's holding people back is the price.

Healthcare would work the same way. Patients could see whichever doctor they want, take whatever medications they want, and get weekly MRIs of their left pinkie just for kicks. They would just have to pay more for some services depending on their choices.

With prices guiding people to make less expensive choices, healthcare costs go down. Our President is firmly committed (to this issue), and has touted 'Health Savings Accounts' or HSAs as part of controlling healthcare costs. With HSAs, people would set up savings accounts that they could use to pay for their medical expenses.

But not everyone is giggling like a teenager who snuck into an 'R' rated movie about Consumer-Driven Healthcare. Opponents point out a few rather important downfalls.

First, we don't have medical services laid out in neat displays with prices hanging by them. There are no banners outside pharmacies saying they'll beat any competitor's price. There are no coupons in the Sunday paper for a free right pinkie MRI with the purchase of a left pinkie MRI. (Not valid with other offers; one coupon per person.) Most people, including many in the healthcare industry, don't know how much services cost. Without being able to compare prices, it is very difficult to choose among different healthcare providers, services, and medications.

Second, unlike pants, paying less for healthcare services, or doing without certain services, doesn't necessarily save money. The middle-aged man who doesn't want to pay $120 for his annual physical and another $80 for a cholesterol check (those numbers are purely made up—I, too, have no idea how much either of those things cost) might be saving $200 a year, but when he has a heart attack and winds up hospitalized with open heart surgery, the cost goes up into the tens of thousands of dollars.

Third, HSAs are fine and dandy for those who have extra money to set aside, but some argue that it is precisely those who don't have the extra money who need the healthcare coverage.

Consumer-Driven Healthcare may or may not be the answer to our healthcare conundrum. Either way, it's a trend that's going to continue to grow. But fret not. There are so many places in our healthcare system to cut costs that it's only a matter of time before Yankee ingenuity grabs this bull by the horns, drags it to its knees, ties it up, slaughters it, chops it into fancy cuts of steak, grills it over an open flame on the prairie and serves it up with a slice of rhubarb pie and a pint of beer. Now that's what I call progress!

Correlation is Not Causation

'Music correlation is not causation', drones the lead singer of 'Soul Coughing', an alternative rock band that combines coffee house poetry with big band base lines and modern beats. That line is one of the few I actually understand. I believe he's referring to people's actions being blamed on the type of music they listen to. For example, if someone is jay-walking while listening to polka music, that should not be grounds for banning polka music as part of a greater jay-walking fighting campaign (not to mention that it would take away one of our precious few remaining excuses for wearing plaid knickers.) The music and the act are correlated, but one is not causing the other. The same thing applies to many things, including some health-related issues. With new research coming out almost daily, it can be helpful to keep in mind which results are correlations, and which are causations.

Let's look at a few examples:

There is a correlation between lightning and thunder. Whenever there is a flash of lightning, there is also the sound of thunder. But lightning does not cause thunder, and thunder does not cause lightning. A separate event, i.e., Zeus becomes angry and hurls a lightning bolt at those who place sub-par gifts at his temple (people should know by now that he likes his lamb shanks medium-rare) causes both lightning *and* thunder. Therefore, we can say that there is a correlation between thunder and lightning, but one does not cause the other.

Another example is winter time and sadness (commonly known as Seasonal Affective Disorder or SAD). For some people, winter time is correlated with feeling sad. It's possible that winter time causes sadness. But perhaps it's the sad feelings that bring about winter time. After all, at Disneyland (the 'happiest place on earth'), winter time is much milder than in most other parts of the country. As further support for this theory, winters at Disney World are even milder than the ones at Disneyland. Since we're on a Disney roll, we can further conclude that Euro-Disney must not be much of a happy place at all!

To further clarify the exact relationship between wintertime and sadness, we can try a few experiments: We can simulate longer days for people who get sad in winter by exposing them to light and seeing if they still develop sadness. To test the converse relationship, we can try to keep everyone happy and see if winter comes anyway.

The first experiment has been done and it worked: Exposing people to light during winter reduced their sadness as demonstrated in that famous episode of 'Northern Exposure' where people were running around in a manic state with those glasses that had light bulbs embedded in them. (Catch the re-run if you missed it. If you can't find the re-run, look for web-cam re-enactments on You Tube by anyone with 'Fleishman' in their screen name.)

The second experiment is carried out annually between Christmas and New Year in the form of a media and social blitz of good feelings. Unfortunately, it never quite reaches the one hundred percent happy mark, so I suppose we'll never know if universal happiness will bring about warmer weather.

So the conclusion from the above research is that, for some people, the shorter days of winter *cause* sadness. But we needed the further research to clarify that link. Therefore, just because two things are occurring together, it doesn't necessarily mean that one is causing the other.

Headlines about research that has shown a correlation tend to include the words 'tied to' or 'linked'. For example, a headline that states, 'Hole-y socks linked to smelly feet', would imply a correlation. But if the headline states, 'Smelly feet found to weaken sock fabric', it could be proof of a causative relationship.

So until someone does research showing that people who don't normally jay-walk start jay-walking when exposed to polka music, I'm going to keep my plaid knickers pressed and clean and will continue to diligently practice my accordion.

Cox-2,
An Affair to Forget

We awoke that brisk fall morning, rolled over in bed, only to find an empty spot next to us. Vioxx was gone.

No note.

No flowers.

No forwarding address.

We remember it like it was about six months ago. We promised ourselves we would never take a Cox-2 again. Sure, we had other suitors. And some of us even went on rebound flings with Celebrex or Bextra, but it just wasn't the same. There were so many unanswered questions. Was it us? Was it something we did?

Then, that balmy late winter afternoon, it was back. We still remember it like it was about three or four weeks ago. (Time gets blurred when your inflammation is uncontrolled.) Vioxx said it was sorry. That it didn't mean to hurt us and it just had some issues it needed to sort out. Something about heart attacks and strokes. We'd like to believe it, but we're not sure. 'After all, we've been hurt before', we say, recalling Rezulin and Baycol.

Yes, the Cox-2 affair does read like a Harlequin novel.

So here we are in the post-Vioxx recall/unrecall era. What happened?

Basically, Vioxx was being a bad boy. (We'll go with the male gender because we are more prone to causing distress . . . and my wife insisted.) All the while he was reducing our pain and inflammation and protecting our guts, he was literally eating away at our brains and our hearts, raising our risk of heart attack and stroke.

When the proverbial intestinal waste hit the proverbial portable ventilation device, Merck, the maker of Vioxx, voluntarily pulled it from the market and the FDA went to work. They reviewed, reviewed, reviewed, and reviewed some more. Then, the advisory committee voted to put it back on the market. The vote was 15-13 with two abstentions. Talk about a close shave!

But the glory days are over. Never again will patients be so eager to take, nor will doctors be so quick to prescribe, Vioxx.

Its cousins, Celebrex and Bextra, have come under similar scrutiny and have been found guilty of the same side effects to varying degrees.

So what is an inflamed and in-pain patient to do? Like those pharmaceutical commercials tell you, 'Talk to your doctor'.

Here's some background to help you on your way:

A long, long, long, long time ago, there was aspirin. It relieved pain. It reduced inflammation. It wasn't a steroid. What would you call such a drug? How about a Non-Steroidal Anti-Inflammatory Drug? How about NSAID for short? How about a cup of coffee while you're at it?

Aspirin, however, had one major flaw. Over time, it burned a hole in some people's stomachs and apparently that's not OK with the average Josephine. That's when Yankee ingenuity gave us a whole slew of other NSAIDs that didn't burn holes as quickly—but could, if they really wanted to. In this family, we have ibuprofen (Motrin, Advil), naprosyn (Aleve), diclofenac (Cataflam), sulindac (Clinoril), piroxicam (Feldene), indomethacin (Indocin) and eight others. (Google 'me-too' drugs.)

Into this void came the Cox-2s. They were different. They came in bright boxes and had cool names that contained the letter 'X'. All the other NSAIDs wanted to hang out with them. What made them so cool was that they did all the things a traditional NSAID did (for those of you not paying attention, that's reducing inflammation and not being a steroid), but they didn't affect the stomach.

And there was much rejoicing in the land!

Were they any stronger than the old NSAIDs? Definitely not. Their only difference was the lack of any harm to the stomach. Also, they cost ten times as much. How much is an intact stomach lining worth to you?

Soon the Cox-2s were a booming business raking in billions yearly until that fateful September when it all came to a grinding, osteoarthritic halt.

So as the crowds disperse, the confetti settles, and the streamers come down, we see ourselves faced with a difficult decision regarding these Cox-2s. What shall we do with them? Do they have a place in our arsenal of pain management?

I'd like to enlist the help of our politicians in answering this one: yes and no.

A Cut Below the Rest

Each election year, nearly one-third of Americans go to the poles to choose a leader for the rest of the country. In the campaign trail leading up to the election, candidates go head-to-head and smear-to-smear over polarizing, hot-button topics like abortion, healthcare, and the death penalty.

But there is one topic that is too hot for any election. Not only do candidates dare not broach it, but the press dare not even ask questions about it. In fact, this issue is so inflammatory that even ordinary people rarely discuss it. The topic is circumcision.

Not being one to back down from controversy (see the scathing chapter on acne herein), I have taken it upon myself to thrust this issue into the spotlight. Prudence be darned!

First, let's define 'circumcision': Circumcision is the removal of the foreskin of the male genitalia which results in exposure of the glans and the corona radiata. The glans is the helmet-looking part at the tip of the penis, and the corona radiata is the edge of the helmet. Corona radiata is either Latin for luminous crown, or it's some type of beer reference. Either way, that's what happens when men get to name body parts.

But I digress.

A circumcision is usually done within the first two weeks of life. Urologists, obstetricians, family physicians and some pediatricians can perform circumcisions.

The American Academy of Pediatrics (AAP) has taken the radical stance of not recommending for or against routine circumcision. After reviewing 40 years of scientific data, and a nice warm cup of hot cocoa, the AAP concluded that even though circumcision does offer some health benefits, those health benefits are not 'significant enough' to justify routine circumcision.

The health benefits of circumcision include, but are not limited to, decreased chance of bladder infections and sexually transmitted diseases.

An uncircumcised child's risk of a bladder infection is 1 in 100; a circumcised child's risk is 1 in 1000. In other words, the risk is reduced from one percent to 0.1 percent. Neither number is terribly alarming. Although, if I were a Pro-Circumcision candidate's campaign manager, I'd have him/her declare in a Pro-Circumcision rally 'Circumcision cuts bladder infection risk tenfold!' That would be just what the crowd would be waiting for to whip them into a voting frenzy.

Circumcision also reduces the risk of sexually transmitted diseases, such as syphilis and HIV. But behavioral factors (i.e., abstinence, condom use, etc.) have a much bigger impact. So if I had left my Pro-Circumcision candidate over some steamy sex scandal (involving misuse of public funds and inappropriate use of personal electronics), I would join the rival Pro-Whole-Penis (PWP) camp and would have the PWP candidate declare at a NASCAR rally, 'Circumcision has a negligible effect on controlling sexually transmitted diseases. Let's focus our efforts on Sex Ed!' (I don't know why, but I envision NASCAR people as being PWPs.)

However, in some African countries, circumcision is being considered as a way of controlling the spread of HIV. If African politics is anything like politics in this country, the Pro-Circumcision people there have their work cut out for them.

So no matter who wins the next election, I don't think either side of the circumcision camp has anything to fear, which is a good thing, considering that there are other issues that need our more immediate attention. Perhaps we can save this fiery debate until all the other issues have been resolved. In the meantime, may we all take pride in our stances on the circumcision issue and at least acknowledge the other side—even though, deep down inside, we know we are more right.

Cut the Cord, Tie the Knot

There is a large discrepancy in fashion choices between men and women. For women, there are blouses, camisoles, halter tops, cardigans, tube tops, flutter sleeve, sleeveless, and three-quarter's sleeve. For men, there are shirts and ties. This discrepancy somehow carries over into contraception. Women have at their disposal pills, shots, patches, vaginal rings, cervical caps, diaphragms, gels, foams, intrauterine devices and surgical sterilization aka 'tube tying'. Men can choose from condoms or a vasectomy.

In order to understand what a vasectomy is, we must first understand what it is that is getting '-ectomy'ed. The 'vas' in 'vasectomy' refers to the 'vas deferens.' In order to understand the vas deferens, we must first understand that, like 'fish', the singular and plural of 'vas deferens' are the same. As in, 'After each vas deferens was cut, both vas deferens were cauterized.' However, this does not mean that a group of vas deferens would be called a 'school.' In fact, we don't have a term for a group of vas deferens because the situation has never come up.

So a vasectomy is removing, aka '-ectomy'ing, the vas deferens. The vas deferns are the tubes that connect the testicles to the urethra. They can be easily felt through the scrotum. They are the hard tubes above each testicle. The vas deferens' job is to move sperm from the testicles to the urethra. The urethra is the large tube that carries forth all emissions from the male nether regions.

When a man goes in for a vasectomy, he lies down on the exam table. The urologist or family physician feels the vas deferens through the scrotum. He/she then numbs the skin with lidocaine, makes a small incision, pulls out the vas deferens through said incision and then cuts the vas deferens. Some physicians remove a segment of the vas, creating a gap between the two ends. Some burn the ends and/or tie them with sutures (a French Knot would be a nice touch). It's like bombing a bridge, trampling the debris with tanks, then washing it all away with a flood. All are measures to prevent the bridge from re-building itself, which the vas deferens have been known to do.

The risks of the procedure are fairly small. There is a very minor risk of bleeding or infection. Some men get a spermatocele, aka ball of sperm, at the spot where the vas is cut. One can imagine the sperm waiting at the site, looking at their watches, tapping their feet, and texting other sperm wondering what the hold-up is. But that would be incorrect. Sperm do not text message.

Almost always, the spermatocele causes no symptoms and needs no treatment.

This brings up a very common question, 'What happens to the sperm that can't get out?' The same thing that happens when a man is abstinent. Sperm have a very short shelf-life. If they sit around too long, they start to get abnormal or die. So the body, after a few days, breaks down the sperm and sells the parts to the testicles. Those parts are used to make more sperm.

As for the patient, everything else stays the same. Sexual function does not change in any way except for shooting 'blanks.' In other words, the mail is still delivered, but the envelopes are empty.

Recovery time from the surgery is relatively quick as well. Men who don't do heavy labor usually get the procedure done on a Friday and, after a weekend with ice and anti-inflammatories, are back on the job on Monday without even walking funny.

So the next time one's flipping through the 'Contraceptives Today' catalog, one can skip the page on men's contraception because nothing will be different. But if a man is absolutely certain he desires no more offspring, the vasectomy is a viable and reliable option that will not diminish one's passion for football or NASCAR, nor will it spur a sudden interest in interior design.

Cuts: An Open or Closed Case

The Third District, 5th Precinct, caddy-corner court summer session is now in session. The Honorable S. Kehl presiding. Please observe the 'No Groaning' sign. This is the case of *Scab v. Bandage*. All rise. Be seated. All rise again. Touch your right toe. Now touch your left toe. Stretch arms over head.

Now that you are warmed up, you may be seated.

-Has the jury reached a verdict?

-Yes we have, your Honor.

-Is the verdict unanimous?

-Yes it is, your Honor.

-Is the verdict anonymous?

-No, your Honor. We are calling it 'Gwendolyn'.

-Is the verdict synonymous?

-Yes. With adjudication, conclusion, and ruling as per *www.thesaurus.com*.

-Proceed.

-We, the jury, find the defendant equally guilty as the prosecutor.

This is the opening of a pilot for a new TV show I've been working on entitled: 'Medical Mayhem—The FDA Files'. It's about prosecutors in the Food and Drug Administration seeking out and bringing to justice various treatment modalities/medications. Each week would be a new case of contrasting approaches to the same problem such as diet vs. exercise for weight loss or counseling vs. medication for depression. (There would be an ongoing side plot about herbal supplements (natraceuticals) and how the prosecutors are powerless to act against them even though natraceuticals cause some Medical Mayhem of their own.)

The pilot is about treating cuts and scrapes. The city is ravaged by a war between rival gangs: Scabbers and Banders.

The Scabbers believe in keeping wounds open to the air so that they form scabs. They argue that forming a scab protects the injured site and keeps it from getting infected. The body then heals the wound from underneath the scab. When the wound is healed, the scab falls off by itself.

Scabbers spray-paint graffiti on city buses that scabs require little effort to maintain and are more durable than bandages.

The Banders, on the other hand, spray-paint graffiti on highway signs that keeping a cut covered with a bandage is best. They arm themselves with tubes of antibiotic ointment and use it in conjunction with bandages.

They argue that bandages work better in areas of the skin that have a lot of movement like elbows, knuckles, and knees. They say that scabs in these areas break whenever the area is moved and that repeats the cycle of pain, bleeding and scabbing. They claim that bandages allow better movement of scraped joints.

As fate would have it (and it often does), a Scabber boy falls in love with a Bander girl. They try to shun their love, but it overwhelms them. They are racked with guilt over betraying their gangs and yet cannot stand to be apart. They thus devise an elaborate scheme to elope involving a trip to the ER, where they are attended by some doctors in *Scrubs* and are taken away on an *Amazing Race* by some *Desperate Housewives* and wind up getting *Lost*.

The episode ends with the Banders and Scabbers realizing that they are both effective in treating cuts and scrapes and that they each have their own unique role to fill. They start cooperating to make their town better by serving dinner to the homeless and raising awareness about the signs and symptoms of an infected cut or scrape. They start visiting parks and beaches in the summertime, informing people that a wound that is hard, hot, red and getting more painful instead of better is suspicious for being infected and needs to be evaluated by a healthcare provider. They clean up their old gang graffiti and instead do art in sanctioned areas using clever slogans like, 'If it's hot, clean it's not'. Or 'If it's oozing, get it checked out, it's the right choosing.'

I think the show has a lot of potential. After all, if they're going to air a re-make of the Bionic Woman . . .

The Danger Within

I couldn't believe the headline of the New York Times today. Some nonsense about the Middle East when I had distinctly informed them well in advance that my daughter had taken her first step. I use the singular of step for a reason: She only took one step. She was standing, took one meaningful, well-planned step, and then—as if to signify that her point had been made—sat down and started to chew on a coaster.

This amazing event seemed to set a ripple across the living room, through the kitchen, up the stairs to the bedrooms and out into the yard. Like so many Disney movies, this ripple had a transformative effect: our quaint abode with its simple, comfortable, if not entirely matching furniture was transformed in an instant to a menacing dungeon with implements of harm at every turn.

How could we live like this? How could we bring a child into this house of destruction and peril?

Our coffee tables' edges and legs seemed to glisten like the blades of so many swords. The wires of the computer and television were creating sparks that seemed to call out our daughter's name. And don't get me started on the stairs which had already, more than once, tried to do us in.

I rushed to the back corner of the bonus room of my mind and started to ruffle through the clutter of papers on the desk. And like so many other times that I had come there looking for something, I found everything else but the item I was looking for: A reading list, a yellow sticky note reminding me to get a gift for my cousin's birthday last week, and some old chewing gum. (I really should put a trash can in there.)

Finally, there it was. Right next to the commemorative pen from my graduation: the 'Childproofing Your House' list. I guess it was time to start working on it. I had gathered the information from observation of friends' houses with children and—of all places—from the Social Security Administration web site, *www.ssa.gov*. It's amazing how many things our government does that I don't know about—both good and not so good.

We needed gates for the stairs, latches for the cabinets and drawers, plugs for the electric outlets, a lock for the toilet lid, foam padding for sharp edges, child-proof covers for door knobs, and netting for the balcony upstairs because the rails were more than six inches apart. The web site also recommended door stops. Apparently, doors are a major cause of amputations in the home. Yikes!

During a trip to the Los Angeles area, I went to a Target store to see what they had. Like the desk in the bonus room of my mind, they seemed to have everything else but child-proofing items. After having traversed all child-related aisles twice, it was time to ask for help. So I asked one of the employees and she directed me to the end of one aisle that had their child-proofing items. It was all rather anti-climactic. I had expected a big sign saying, 'Protect your child!' or some sort of propaganda to make me feel like a bad parent if I didn't buy a certain product. But no, these products were just sitting there, rather non-descript. They seemed to know their own importance and thus didn't feel the need to make a lot of noise. Much to my surprise, I was able to buy most everything I needed from that aisle-end.

As of this writing, I have opened one of the gates and inspected it. All the parts are present and I have a vague sense of how to install it. The rest of the items are still in their packages safely sitting on the garage floor where they can cause no harm (except to me as I trip over them getting to the car). I've learned over the last week, however, that these things don't install themselves.

One more item on the child-proofing list that didn't require purchasing was turning down the temperature on the water heater to 120 degrees. All water heaters have a dial to control the temperature. Setting the dial to 120 degrees gives parents more time to get to the child before she gets burned when she wanders into the bathroom and turns on the hot water.

So I hope to have our living space child-proofed before my daughter graduates from college. Of course, by then, we'll be preparing for grandchildren so I might as well keep them up. In so doing, I hope to somewhat tame the beast that is our living space.

Down the 'Donut Hole'

There are a few signs of changing seasons that are present even in the most temperate climates: The days get shorter, the temperatures dip, and some trees lose their leaves. Now we can add a third sign: some seniors go off of their medications.

This is thanks to the 'donut hole' in Medicare part D. The masterminds of the Medicare Modernization Act (MMA) who brought us part D must have thought that seniors would identify with deep-fried, doughy pastries. Either that or they were on their low-carb diets at the time and the carb-craving beast inside them was raging. Either way, there is a gap in medication coverage for part D subscribers. Medication is covered until $2400, at which point nothing is covered until the expenses add up to $3600. That lack of coverage is called the 'donut hole'.

So a senior caught in the donut hole has two options: pay for medication or do without. Those who choose to pay tend to go to the same pharmacies they've used all along, never stopping to wonder if the same medication would be less expensive elsewhere. After all, buying medication is not like buying a car—or is it?

It might not be in Canada or France where drug prices are regulated. But in the United States, pharmacies operate the same as any other business. They buy items wholesale, and mark it up to cover additional costs and make a profit. Some pharmacies have a higher markup than others.

I came to this stark realization about a year ago when I received a call from a patient I had seen that had no insurance. In treating her acid reflux, I prescribed ranitidine, a generic antacid that tends to go for about $13 for a month's supply. I spoke to her a few days later and she informed me that she had not gotten the prescription filled because the pharmacy was going to charge her over fifty dollars!

I was surprised, dismayed, and confused—enough to give *me* acid reflux, but I knew where I was *not* going to buy my reflux medication. So I called the pharmacy in question to inquire about it and got an answer that was very political. Some words were exchanged, but I hung up the phone knowing nothing more than when I started.

This pharmacy was a national chain that usually has great deals on many items ranging from shaving cream to athletic tape to wine-in-a-box (all essential ingredients for a party). Yet some locally owned and operated pharmacies charge much less for the same medication.

As it turns out, the pharmacy that has the smallest markup and, as a result, the least expensive medication is the same establishment that brought us barrel-sized containers of licorice, giant chocolate cakes, and two-pound bags of M&Ms (more essential ingredients for a party) all for under fifteen dollars. That's right! The establishment in question is none other than Costco. The best part is that one need not be a card-carrying member to reap the benefits of their great drug prices.

Since the pharmacies are free to adjust their prices, consumers who have no insurance or find themselves in the donut hole are also free to shop around and compare prices between pharmacies. The internet makes that search very easy. For those without internet connection, the phone book can be very helpful.

Let's look at a few examples: lisinopril, a generic blood pressure medication, costs $11.99 at the big national chain and only $5 at Costco. Lovastatin, a generic cholesterol medication, costs $22.99 at the chain and only $13.13 at Costco. To be fair, brand name medications tend to run about the same in both places.

So perhaps pharmacies will become like ski resorts with an 'off' season and an 'on' season. Perhaps we'll hear radio advertisements for 'season opener' or 'Out of the Donut Hole' specials in January. Why not throw in a family deal of four lift tickets with each prescription filled? The possibilities are endless!

A Drug by Any Other Name
(Would Cost Half as Much)

As Consumer-Driven Healthcare (see chapter herein) spreads its wings and glides over this great land, like the great bald eagle of liberty, one mark that it has already left on our newly washed cars is its effect on prescription drug coverage.

Virtually anyone who has ever filled a prescription realizes that brand name medications cost a lot more than generic ones. Most people know that some medications are available in generic form while others are not. Few people know *why* some medications are available in generic form, while others are not.

The generic name of a medication is the name the scientists give it as they're discovering/inventing the drug. It typically gives some information about the chemical structure of the drug. Generic names tend to be long, difficult to pronounce, and rhyme with other medications in the same family. For example, the generic name for all the drugs in the 'statin' family—a group of cholesterol-reducing medications that includes Lipitor—ends in 'statin', i.e., lovastatin, simvastatin, atorvastatin, and rosuvastatin.

Brand names, on the other hand, are peppy. They invoke certain feelings. They're easy to remember. And that's the name the inventing company gives the drug for marketing purposes.

Let's follow the story of a fictitious drug to see how the process works:

There's a lonely molecule floating in a beaker in some lab somewhere that can cure obesity. This drug will be the 'magic pill' everyone's been waiting for. Let's call it 'Phil' for starters. As scientists experiment with Phil and learn more about him, they give him a name which partly has to do with his chemical structure. Since Phil is a protein and he has a divalent sodium bond trans ring with a carboxy aldehyde group in the seven position, they decide to call him sodicarbaldehydroxyvalentelin. This is Phil's generic name.

At this point, Drug Company X quickly becomes involved. They take Phil, make him into a pill form and start doing human experiments. As experiments confirm that Phil indeed is the 'magic pill' for obesity, the marketing department of Company X starts developing ideas on how to sell Phil. They are the 'extreme makeover' people of the pharmaceutical world. First step is to come up with a new name. Sodicarbaldehydroxyvalentelin is difficult to remember and, frankly, rather drab. They want a name that's snappy, something that will be easy to remember and that people will associate with being thin and feeling happy. They come up with 'Graelin'. It rhymes with thin and has the gra—prefix derived from gracilis which is Latin for slim. It also sort of sounds like 'gay' (meaning happy). This is Phil's brand name.

For the next ten years, it's party time at Drug Company X. Since they were the ones to develop Phil, the law allows them to be the only company to manufacture and sell Phil. The company goes on a selling spree: They send sales representatives to doctors' offices in full force, armed with medication samples, pens, note pads, laser pointers and belt buckles all saying 'Graelin'. They fly guest speakers across the country and down the street to tout its merits. They book a spot on 'Oprah.' They run advertisements in prime time showing shiny, happy, skinny people holding hands and walking on the beach in skimpy outfits.

And Phil does well. He alone brings in billions of dollars a year in revenue for Drug Company X. Phil is 'blockbuster' drug.

But all too soon, the ten years are up. Then other manufacturers start making Phil. They can't use the name 'Graelin', but it's the same old Phil everyone knows and loves. As more generic companies start making Phil, Phil becomes cheaper and cheaper and more accessible to the public.

Thus is the life span of a drug in the American marketplace. So the next time you get a prescription filled, realize that if it's something advertised on television, chances are there's no generic available. However, if it's something that's at least ten years old, you're in luck. Now we can all wash our cars in peace.

E. Coli Are Us

The last outbreak of E.coli in spinach has given new armament to some children's pleas to be excused from consuming this green, leafy vegetable. It makes me wonder what Popeye would say. (Aside from his standard 'I yam whadayyam'.)

If Popeye were a conspiracy theorist (and if you don't think he is, then they've gotten to you, too), he'd find a babysitter for Swee'pea, call a meeting with Olive Oyl, that hamburger-eating guy (who still hasn't paid even though it's well past Tuesday), and maybe even Bluto, and take a long, suspicious, conspiratorial look at the fast-food industry. One of the basic principles of investigative work, so I hear, is to consider who would benefit from the crime. This one's a no-brainer: Not only does the fast-food industry create a diversion from its own previous difficulties with contamination, but it drives more people away from vegetables and possibly into the arms of their local fast-food chain.

But there is more to E.coli than meets the eye. A closer look will show us how E.coli is very much like us.

We live on the planet Earth (or so NASA would have us believe). E.coli lives in organisms that live on planet Earth. Most humans are kind, peace-loving people who want nothing more than to live in harmony with the world around them. Most E.coli are a normal part of the human colon and want nothing more than to live their lives in peace and harmony with all the other bacteria that live in the human large intestine.

But not all humans are your standard peace-loving variety. Some choose to follow paths of violence and destruction. Similarly, not all E.coli are the human-intestine-living-and-loving-it variety. Some can cause illness if ingested, though I don't think it's of their own choosing.

One such variety is the infamous O157:H7 strain of E.coli. A 'strain' is the bacterial equivalent of a dog breed. I don't know what the O157:H7 stands for. But I do know that it's fun to say and can make someone sound really knowledgeable. Look for opportunities in casual conversation to throw it in. For example, you could say, 'I went to the auto expo last weekend and the new Audi prototype O157:H7 looks really cool!'

But I digress.

E.coli O157:H7 can contaminate foods. And as recent events have shown us, this outlaw of the E.coli community never met a food it didn't like. Once ingested, the O157:H7 can release a toxin. This toxin can cause diarrhea and abdominal pain. In some cases, the diarrhea can be bloody. Generally, there is no fever.

Most of the time, the body's defenses fight off the infestation and life goes back to normal in the colon. The music starts anew, the party conversation crescendos back to pre-infestation levels, and the spleen resumes its litany of complaints about the noise, stating he 'has to go to work tomorrow'. (We all know the spleen hasn't held a job for years.)

One of the possible complications of diarrhea caused by E.coli O157:H7 is dehydration. Some people can get so dehydrated that they do not survive the illness. Most at risk are the elderly, the very young, and those with weakened immune systems. Fluids through the vein can help fight dehydration. Interestingly, antibiotics are not used because they might actually wind up making the infection worse which can lead to kidney failure and the need for dialysis.

Fortunately, our good friend 'heat' can take care of the bad E.coli before we ingest it. Cooking meats and vegetables thoroughly at temperatures above 155 degrees F. can kill off the E.coli in food and save a lot of trouble.

So Popeye should be safe with canned spinach since it tends to be well-cooked. Perhaps he and Bluto can use this opportunity to reconcile their differences. Now, if we could only get him to stop smoking . . . .

Expecting the Expected

As my wife and I prepared for the impending birth of our first child, we drafted a birth plan which I suppose is the equivalent of drafting a constitution for the moon. Part of our birth plan was music and so we set upon burning some CDs. Here are some songs that my wife promptly vetoed:

'King of Pain' by The Police
'Hurt So Good' by John Mellencamp
'I Gotta Get Through This' by Daniel Bettingfield

These songs *were* included:

'Under Pressure', by Queen and David Bowie
'Push It' by Sallt 'n' Peppa
'I'm Coming Out', by Big Lady K

The other part of our birth plan was an epidural. We already knew that the epidural would be a wondrous, magical thing, but we didn't quite realize how magical and wondrous it would be until the dreaded 'back labor' kicked in. (Until then, I thought back labor was what I did when I spent an entire weekend, using various manual and power tools and an excavation permit, digging up the root stump of the giant cactus that used to be in our front yard. Apparently, adult cacti actually fuse their roots with the planet core. But I digress.)

But watching my wife go up on her toes every three minutes and mutter words that would make Eminem blush has put things in new perspective.

I'd heard from other friends who had gone through the birthing process that the anesthesiologist aka Epidural Guy was the most welcomed face they'd ever seen. I now wholeheartedly agree.

My wife curled her back and held it for a good 30 minutes weathering wave after wave of soul-crushing, back-breaking, deity-invoking contractions just to provide an optimal target area for the anesthesiologist—or as we like to call him, Dr. THANK GOD YOU'RE HERE! DO SOMETHING!!

I have known some people who have looked down and even feared the epidural. Certainly, the thought of having a needle inserted through the back, pumping medication directly into your spinal cavity may not sound very inviting to everyone. I remember vividly when asked in our 'Preparing for Childbirth' class, 'How many people know they want an epidural?' My wife was the only woman of the 13 couples attending who raised her hand.

Some people want to have a natural childbirth experience, free of any medication. Others fear that the epidural could be harmful to the mother or baby. The epidural, as the name suggests, is 'epi' to the 'dura', meaning outside the sheath that covers the spine. The anesthesiologist inserts a needle through a tiny space between the vertebrae—the bony blocks of the spine—and inserts a tiny rubber tube that sits outside the sheath covering of the spine. Then medication is slowly infused into the area around the spine. The result is that the pelvis and legs become numb. Contractions become much less painful and that makes for a happier laboring mother and a father without crushed hand bones.

The epidural, relatively speaking, is quite low risk. There is a very small risk of bleeding or infection. There is also a very, very small risk of headache, if the needle goes beyond the covering of the spine.

As far as the baby's concerned, nothing much is different. The medication does not get into the mother's blood stream and therefore does not affect the baby. Sometimes the contractions slow down after an epidural, as was the case with my wife. But with time, the contractions start up again and you're back on the labor train. The anesthesiologist at my wife's labor described labor without an epidural like getting 'a root canal without Novocain.' I'm not sure I would take it that far. After all, women have not been having root canals on their own for millions of years. But the fact remains that with modern medicine, we have a very good option for pain control during birth. While certainly not a requirement, it is a viable option. (And the husband can go on to a career of playing the piano with undamaged hands, if he so wishes!)

Extract the Badness

I recently ran into an old hypothetical friend. Her name is Juicy Juicerson—JJ for short. But don't call her short—she's very sensitive about her height. She was wearing her usual mall stroll outfit: tight low-rider jeans that made her waist bulge out like the marshmallow part of a s'more and an even tighter t-shirt with the word 'juicy' written across the chest. She had gotten her hair feathered which framed her long face nicely and softened her sharp features.

She started talking about her new passion, 'juicing'. With a name such as hers I suppose it was inevitable. She went on and on about how healthy it was and how much better she felt. How it was 'natural' and how much time it saved her. She invited me over for a juicing party.

I arrived at her hypothetical downtown apartment twenty minutes late. That's my rule for hypothetical parties: arrive twenty minutes late. Not so late that you miss out on prime drinking and not so soon that people think you're desperate. There were people wall to wall. She had six juicers going at the same time. The place sounded like the inside of my mouth during my last dental visit. Everyone had brought their favorite items to juice. There were the standards, such as oranges and apples, less common items, such as melons, carrots, and strawberries, and exotic items, like star fruit, mangos, and radishes. The disposal was filled with pulp and everyone had a glass filled with colorful liquid.

Someone shoved a maroon-beige, clumpy liquid with tan streaks in my face and told me to 'drink it!' Flashing back to my college days, I tilted my head back, took a big gulp, gagged, coughed, and spilled half of it down the front of my brand new Armani sweater. (I always dress up for hypothetical parties. Did I mention my shoes were vintage Nine West?) It tasted like a mixture of the farmer's market on a hot day, olive oil, and plastic.

After having two glasses of I'm-not-sure-what, I was done. I cordially thanked JJ and started to walk home. I was in no condition to drive. As I strolled along, I thought to myself that I should call JJ more often.

I also thought about the juicing experience. These people were downright fanatical in their belief.

So I decided to do some research on my own to test the validity of some of JJ's claims. After all, one shouldn't be so quick to trust the judgment of a hypothetical friend—especially one as eccentric as JJ.

I decided to compare the healthiness of juices, starting with the world-renowned, named-after-the-county-in-Southern-California orange. One orange has 62 calories and 3.1 grams of fiber. One cup of orange juice has 112 calories and 0.5 grams of fiber. Nearly twice the sugar and only 16 percent of the fiber—not so good. How about the always-a-bridesmaid-never-a-bride member of the fruit juice world, the apple? One apple has 81 calories and 3.7 grams of fiber. One cup of apple juice has 117 calories and 0.2 grams of fiber. A virtual home run in the sugar to fiber ratio! (Google 'glycemic index'.)

How about the naturalness of juicing? I went to the store and bought double portions of ingredients for a hypothetical concoction: apple-mango-orang-erine. But they didn't have mango so I settled for apple-orang-erine-nana. When I was finished, I placed my juice glass next to the bowl of fruit. In the bowl, I had fruit just as the trees had made them. In the glass was the result of my mangling of said fruit and extracting the fiber and some vitamins and concentrating the sugars into a liquid form. That's two strikes against JJ. She was not going to take this very well.

Next I decided to tackle the time factor. I measured the time it took me to peel and seed the fruit, take out the juicer, assemble the juicer, juice the fruit, disassemble the juicer, clean it and put it away, and drink the juice. I compared it to the time it took to just eat the fruit straight. It was a close call. A difference of a few minutes in favor of juicing. But certainly nothing to write home about.

I had realized that JJ was not accomplishing what she was hoping to accomplish by juicing. If anything, she was only contributing to further bulging at her waist-line from the high glycemic index of the juices. Yet, I didn't know how to bring it up to her without hurting her feelings or dissuading her from a healthy lifestyle altogether. This could easily send her into a five-day brownie-eating binge, if her past record was anything to go by.

So I sat down at the computer and stared at the blinking cursor at the upper left corner of the screen. I would write, highlight, delete, write, highlight, delete for what seemed like hours. Finally, I put together a letter that I thought brought all the points to her attention without being judgmental and hopefully without dampening her enthusiasm. I printed it on my best stationery and signed it with my favorite pen. I then folded it neatly, put it in an envelope, wrote her address with my mini-calligraphy pen which never made my writing look like a box cover, and put my kitty cat return label on it. I put on a left-over Christmas stamp (JJ was a Christmas fanatic), and placed the letter in the shredder. Better to keep a hypothetical friend than ruin their juicing parties!

Feel the Burn

There are many things that make Carpinteria unique: abundant avocado orchards, the fact that 85 percent of the town's population is related to one another by blood or marriage, and the distinction of having the 'World's Safest Beach'. 'Safe' can mean so many things. Perhaps it means that there is very little crime on the beach. Maybe it means there are no shark attacks. Or possibly it means that one can make it to second base without getting tagged by the ball. (That is strictly a baseball reference.) But the one thing that not even Carpinteria's beach is safe from is the sun and, by extension, sunburns. Admittedly, if they extended the avocado orchards to the beach, that could provide adequate shade and a healthy snack. Then we could also claim that the beach is safe from low levels of good cholesterol (HDL) because of the stanols in the avocados.

But I digress.

So even in Carpinteria, people can get sunburned. A sunburn is no different than any other burn. Whether the heat comes from the sun or from leaving one's hand under a heat lamp all day pretending it's a lizard, the end result it the same: the skin gets inflamed which leads to more blood flow which makes the skin warm and more sensitive to touch which leads to people walking around like the Michelin Tire man. There are many ways to prevent sunburns. Sunscreens can be very helpful. But, in actuality, a sunscreen only delays a sunburn. If we think of sunrays as baseballs being hurled at us from space, a sunscreen would be a batter standing over us hitting them back. ('Batter' meaning someone who swings a bat, not uncooked cake. Although the latter could also work and, on a hot enough day, provide dessert.)The better the batter, the fewer the balls that will get through. But even with the best batter, eventually enough balls will get through to burn us.

Sunscreens come with an SPF rating. The higher the rating, the higher the protection. The number of the SPF means how much longer it would take for the skin to burn compared to using no sunscreen at all. So if one would burn in twenty minutes, using a sunscreen with SPF 10 would delay the burn ten times, or up to 200 minutes. While that may seem like a long time (over three hours), those times are determined in a controlled laboratory setting where subjects are shielded from wind and sweat, and all the lab techs wear long coats and glasses so as not to induce sweating in the subjects. But in the real world, water, wind and sweat all decrease the effectiveness of the sunscreen.

Since sunscreens only delay sunburns, the key to keeping skin safer from the sun is limiting sun exposure. Spending fifteen minutes of every hour in the shade is a good rule of thumb.

Other modes of sun protection include wide-brimmed hats and long-sleeved shirts. These items also have SPF ratings that they may or may not display. So it is possible to get burned using hats and long-sleeved shirts but it will likely take reading a Tom Clancy novel (including the entire 215-page description of the mini-fridge in a nuclear submarine's captain's quarters.) This is why one must read Sue Grafton novels: they're fast paced, easy to read, and better for your skin! They are also a great way to review the alphabet up to letter U.

Once a sunburn has occurred, the treatment is like any other burn. Anti-inflammatories like ibuprofen can help heal the skin. The increased heat from the burn and the increased blood flow can dry out the skin, adding to the discomfort. Moisturizers can help soothe these symptoms.

But if the worst thing that became of a sunburn was a trip to the local pharmacy for some ibuprofen and lotion, most people could live with that. The greater concern about sunburns is the increased risk of skin cancer. In the Marvel Universe, the ultraviolet rays of the sun damage skin cell DNA creating the ability to generate surfable waves in August. Here, in the real world, damaged DNA in skin cells makes them more likely to become cancerous. The more sunburns one has, the higher the risk of skin cancer. 'Blistering' sunburns are especially risky since the deeper layers of the skin are damaged.

So as we enjoy these sunny days in Carpinteria, we can leave home the shark suit and taser. But by bringing an umbrella, a wide-brimmed hat, a long-sleeved shirt and sunscreen of SPF 15 or higher, we can say with confidence that we have truly spent the day at the 'World's Safest Beach'.

Fire in the Sky

Well, it's happened. In spite of your best intentions, it's happened. You wore the wide-brimmed hat. You spent fifteen minutes of every hour in the shade. You wore sunscreen SPF 15 or higher and re-applied after going in the water. And yet, here you are, with the family gathered around you, marshmallows extended on sticks, exchanging ghost stories while basking in the warmth that radiates from you like an old-fashioned Franklin stove.

What is a sun-burnt person to do?

First and foremost, do take time to credit yourself for doing everything right. Had you not exercised good sun protection, you could be worse off than you are now.

Next, let's understand the problem: A sunburn is just like any other burn. Two things determine how much a burn will burn: temperature and time. Immersing the body in a Jacuzzi that has been heated to 100 degrees most likely will not cause a burn, even if one sits in it for hours. But putting your outstretched hand on a hot barbecue grill while trying to adopt a cool pose to impress the girl next door can cause a burn in seconds—both physically and emotionally.

Burns are classified by degrees depending on how deep the burn goes. Let's take the burn elevator to the underground parking lot. (And hope we remember where we parked the silvadine-mobile.) Keep in mind this elevator only goes down!

1st floor (aka first degree): Irritation of the very top layer of the skin. Here you'll find redness, swelling, pain, assorted men's and women's footwear, beauty and fragrance, and juniors clothing.

2nd floor (aka second degree): Irritation of deeper layers of the skin. This floor has all the amenities of the first floor, but also includes blister formation, bedding and furniture. Sorry, no scars here.

3rd floor (aka third degree): Irritation of the entire skin layer and some of the fat and blood vessels underneath. Here you will also find damaged nerves which can mean no pain. Visit the fine china and jewelry department located behind the handbag and accessories display.

Using our handy guide, we can see that most sunburns tend to be first degree (unless they blister, in which case they would be second degree). So what can we do about it?

First and foremost is avoiding further irritation of the already irritated skin. The same way that it would be unwise for a zookeeper to eat a ham sandwich in front of a tiger on its 'fasting' day, it would be unwise to further burn a skin that is already burned.

Second is giving the heat trapped in the skin an escape route. Burns are considered 'dynamic' injuries. This means that not only do they give great lectures, but they can also continue to worsen even when the source of heat is removed.

Consider the climactic battle scene between Count Dooku and Yoda in Star Wars, Episode II. Count Dooku launches a Force-generated lightning bolt at Yoda. Yoda gathers the lightning in his three-digited hand. The ball of Force lightning undulates in Yoda's hand. It must be given a place to go so Yoda chooses to launch it back at Count Dooku.

Heat that has been transferred to the skin works much in the same way. Once the heat is absorbed by the skin, it has to go somewhere. Some of it goes out through the skin, but some of it continues to progress deeper into the skin, causing more injury.

Therefore, it is important to give the heat a place to go. Placing something cool, like a cold (not frozen) piece of steak or some cool water, on the skin gives the heat a very desirable target.

Ibuprofen (Advil, Motrin) can help with the inflammation and moisturizers can help with comfort.

So, just as we would with drinks on the town, let's enjoy the abundant summer sun responsibly. Let's be diligent in our sun protection, and if we should be unlucky enough to get a burn, let's hope we find everything we need in the shoe department.

The Flu-Man Cometh

The flu season arrives. As usual, there was no grand ceremony, no champagne, and no ribbon cutting—just people feeling lousier than they thought possible, aching in places they wish they didn't have, and shaking so much that the neighbors come asking them to make martinis.

In fact, I believe the 'Dementors' in the Harry Potter books/movies weren't sucking people's souls out; they were giving them the flu!

For those of you not familiar with the boy wizard's adventures, the 'Dementors' are floating figures, dressed in tattered black-hooded hand-me-downs from the grim reaper. They float along, freezing the landscape, killing plant life, and making people feel very cold. People describe feeling like they'd 'never be happy again.' If that's not the flu, I don't know what is.

Once touched by a flu Dementor, people can get high fevers (up to 105 degrees), intense body aches, sore throat, cough, and headache. Often, first-timers are left wondering what happened. What kind of cold is this?

The truth is that the flu is quite different from the common cold. Although the two have overlapping symptoms, it can be fairly easy to tell them apart—especially for someone who has experienced the flu.

Perhaps the most important difference between the flu and the common cold is fever and body aches.

The common cold doesn't typically cause fever. The flu, on the other hand, almost always causes a fever, frequently to the point of causing the patient to shiver. People describe this as having 'the chills'. For those who have never experienced 'the chills', it's the sensation of being so cold that nothing can heat you up. People put on jackets over sweatshirts and bury themselves under a small mountain of blankets while eating hot soup and *still* can't stop shaking.

The common cold rarely causes body aches and when it does it's rather mild. The flu has intense body aches that come on very quickly, usually overnight or within a few hours. Patients feel as if they've slept in a trash compactor.

Both the cold and the flu can cause sore throat and headache, but the flu tends to do a much better job of it.

The cough with the flu tends to be 'dry', whereas the cough from a cold can have 'phlegm.'

I, personally, have experienced the flu only once—and I intend to keep it that way. Every year when the flu vaccine is released, I rush to the front of the line, shoving aside small children and old ladies with walkers to ensure that I get my vaccine first (and my sticker and sugar-free lollipop, too).

For those who have had the misfortune of catching the flu, there are a few prescriptions that can help. Each carries its own risks and restrictions. They are most effective when taken within 48 hours of the start of symptoms. Ibuprofen in high enough doses can greatly help with the body aches, fever, and sore throat. Cough suppressants with codeine can help control night-time cough and facilitate sleep.

So for those of you who have been touched by the flu 'Dementor', hang in there. Talk to your healthcare provider about medications that might help. And rest assured that the sun will come out, the chill will go away, and happiness will return. Once that happens, consider getting a flu vaccine next year. It's the greatest 'Patronus Charm' we have to fight this 'Dementor'.

(*Author's Note: The flu vaccine is not actually a 'charm'. It is a shot. On second thought, it is administered with a wand of sorts and it is free-flowing like the charms in the movies, so maybe it is a charm after all! Never mind.*)

Forget the Doctor,
Get the Toolbox!

Frogs have gotten a bum rap. They don't give people warts. *People* give people warts.

Warts are caused by viruses. The virus gets on the skin, infects the very top layer and causes it to become thick and rough, prompting people to seek ways to get rid of it.

There are many home remedies that people have tried with varying success rates. I won't mention any of them here mainly because I don't remember any of them (although I vaguely recall hearing something about eye of newt and three hairs from a Shetland pony), but also because some of them can cause more harm than good.

In the medical setting, we can use liquid nitrogen, salicylate paper—commonly known as 'acid paper', or blistering agents, again with varying success rates.

To this regimen of varyingly successful regimens we can now add duct tape. That's right, good old fix-everything-now-including-warts duct tape. It's quite simple. Cover the wart with a small piece of duct tape (any color will do) for six days straight. On the seventh day, remove the tape, soak the wart in water for twenty minutes and rub with a pumice stone. (A pumice stone is a rough rock used on skin and is available in most drug stores.) Then wait 24 hours. If the wart is still there, repeat the cycle. The cycle can be repeated up to two months. The success rate is about 75 percent, which is better than most other treatment modalities.

How it works is anyone's guess. I don't think Mr. Duct purposefully designed his tape to be endowed with anti-wart properties. My personal suspicion is that it works much in the same way that any other wart treatment works, i.e., it irritates the skin enough to draw the body's attention. The immune system does the rest.

In fact, if you do *nothing* to a wart, your body *will* eventually get rid of it, just like any other viral infection. The problem is that the wart virus lives in the very top layer of skin where there isn't a lot of blood flow and so it takes a while, about five to ten years, for the body to catch on that there's an infection. Most people don't want to wait that long.

A few provisos on the duct tape regimen. It doesn't seem to work so well for 'plantar warts', which are warts on the soles of feet and actually have nothing to do with plants. (Another bum rap). Also, I would advise against using it on the face. Sure, Batman's sidekick, Robin, made fabric on the face hip, but I wouldn't want to extend that fashion statement to include duct tape.

So the next time you see someone with a tiny piece of duct tape on their skin, you'll know their secret: they've read this book, too.

Fungus in our Midst

This is the story of five little piggies. You know the one: where one goes to the market because he's tired of getting nagged by the second one for never doing his fair share of house chores. The second one stays home, yet again, while the first piggy takes a good three hours to get a dozen eggs and a pound of Red Delicious apples when the market is just five minutes away. The third piggy, with her overly dyed and styled hair, strange tattoos, and pierced snout, ruminates in the corner eating meat much to the disgust of the rest of the vegetarian piggy family. Piggy the fourth refuses to eat because 'there are pigs being eaten all over the world, mom!' And the fifth piggy runs crying to his room because he's ashamed of how his toes look. He says they're all yellow and thick and curled up and just 'gross'.

While in-depth discussion of the family dynamics involved in this piggy family is beyond the scope of this chapter, the particular problem of the fifth little piggy is not. He suffers from toenail fungus. Medically speaking, it is called 'onychomycosis', pronounced 'oooooodon'tlookatmyfeet.'

The fifth little piggy's problem with self-consciousness becomes even more pronounced during the summer months when everyone's toes are put on display. He chooses to get strange looks from others for wearing closed-toe shoes at the beach rather than risk facing the reaction he imagines they will have if they were to see his toes as they are.

Fungus in the toenails usually starts with fungus on the feet, aka 'Athlete's Foot'. 'Athlete's Foot', in turn, tends to occur in feet that get warm and sweaty. (It seems that we're not the only organisms that enjoy warm, humid environs.) The heat and humidity sends the fungus into amorous raptures and a reproductive frenzy (wish we had *that* in common, too!) causing the skin on the feet to become red and start peeling.

Once the fungus is established on the skin, it makes the jump to the toenail. Perhaps they take a vote to see who gets to go to this 'New World'. Perhaps some fungi become disgruntled with the overcrowding and lack of employment on the skin and decide to risk it all and journey to the toenails.

Once the select few fungi arrive at the toenail, they find little resistance from the native immune cells (due to low blood flow under the nails) and quickly establish colonies. Here, they are safe from any athlete's foot treatments that wreak havoc on the fungi on the skin. Perhaps the newly arrived fungi on the toenail feel it is their destiny to occupy the entire nail and all the other nails of the foot.

The result of this fungal manifest destiny is that toenails get thick and discolored. But much to their credit, the fungi in the toenails are quite content with simply trashing the place. They don't cause any other symptoms or any other health problems. But the appearance is enough to cause plenty of mental anguish for Piggy the Fifth.

So when Piggy the Fifth goes to see his veterinarian, he's in for a rude awakening. Given that toenail fungus doesn't cause any health problems, his insurance company won't cover the treatment. The only treatment available is by prescription. He would need to take the medication for three months and it would cost him about $300 per month.

The big question Piggy the Fifth needs to ask himself is, how much does the toenail fungus really bother him? The rest of the piggy family, being shocked and dismayed at the conundrum in which Piggy the Fifth finds himself, decide to keep their feet cool and dry and treat skin fungus as soon as it starts. Perhaps that can keep them from having even more fungus among them.

(*Editor's Note:* Do pigs even *have* toenails?)

The Fuss is Pertussis

Many illnesses have aliases. They have a scientific name that scientists use. They also have a common name that everyone else uses. Healthcare providers use both names depending on their audience. If they're speaking at a scientific convention or trying to help someone stuck on a crossword puzzle, they'll use the scientific name and insist the crossword is wrong if their answer doesn't fit. If they're addressing patients, they tend to use the common name unless the patient is a scientist—or looks like a scientist.

Often the common name is much more descriptive than the scientific name. For example, 'heart attack' conveys danger, urgency and damage to the heart. The scientific name for a heart attack is 'myocardial infarction' which sounds like an elite social event as in, 'I'm having a myocardial infarction at the club this afternoon. You should stop by.'

Whooping cough is the common name for an infection caused by the bacteria *Bordatella Pertussis*. Scientists refer to it as 'Pertussis,' but 'whooping cough' is much more descriptive. The name comes from the classic symptom of the disease where patients have coughing fits that force all the air out of their lungs and when they take a deep, forceful breath in, they make a 'whoop' sound. It is the same sound the movie hero/heroine makes when they break through the water surface after rescuing their nemesis' pet from a drowning vehicle only to have their nemesis mock and berate them for their compassion.

But I digress.

Whooping cough is a tricky entity for many reasons. First is that the early stages of the infection are just like the common cold with runny nose, cough, and body aches so it's very difficult to tell who has just a cold and who has whooping cough. Unfortunately, this is also the stage at which it is most contagious. After a week or two, the coughing fits and the 'whoop' start. But like most 'classic' symptoms, the 'whoop' isn't always present. So by the time we suspect that someone has whooping cough, it's already too late to stop the spread.

Second, it is most dangerous to newborns and infants under six months of age. Parents, siblings and other caregivers transmit the illness via infectious droplets. Infectious droplets are the drops of mucus that are expelled when one sneezes or coughs or gets punched in slow motion in a Rocky movie. Quite often, adults who take care of children don't even know they have whooping cough since they have symptoms of what seems like a common cold.

There is a vaccine to protect infants from whooping cough. It is administered at two, four and six months of life. But that leaves infants under two months of age. They are too young to receive the vaccine, and too young for the antibiotics commonly used to treat whooping cough. For them, prevention is key. Since they can't get vaccinated, the next best thing is for all their household contacts, children and adults, to get vaccinated. This is why it is recommended that all adults and teenagers get a whooping cough booster shot. This is also why it is very important to cover one's cough, especially around infants.

So in whooping cough we have a nemesis who is well disguised. It is poised to strike before we know it. And it likes to go after our most vulnerable members. But with due diligence, covering our infectious droplets, and making sure that everyone who *can* get vaccinated *is* vaccinated, we can cut off this nemesis at the pass. (And we would still rescue its pet from a sinking vehicle. Because that just the kind of heroes and heroines we are.)

More information on whooping cough is available at the Center for Disease Control website, *www.cdc.gov*, complete with harrowing audio recordings of adults and children with whooping cough, guaranteed to be sure you don't fall asleep while reading the relevant information.

Good-Bye, Low-Carb;
Hello, Bariatric Surgery

The Atkins Corporation has filed for bankruptcy. How is that for the ultimate symbol of the end of an era! I suppose it was fun while it lasted. Bun-less bacon cheeseburgers, pork chops, and beef jerky dipped in nacho cheese sauce is not a bad way to diet. But apparently it's difficult to sustain.

The shunned, ostracized carbohydrate is peeking its head out of its hiding place to find a hungry public awaiting it with open arms. Welcome back, carb! Oh, how we've missed you! Pass the sugar-covered cotton candy dipped in caramel!

This means the hunt is back on for the next hot thing in weight control. With obesity being the epidemic that it is, and all the money that can be made from an effective treatment, I'm sure this will not be the last we've heard of weight-control remedies.

Bariatric surgery is a current hot topic. It works. The pounds drop off like antidepressants jumping out of a scientologist's medicine cabinet. In fact, people lose weight so fast that they sometimes end up with skin flaps that need to be removed surgically. People's diabetes and high blood pressure can be cured. And, at least in the short run (two to three years), people seem to keep off most of what they lose.

There are many different bariatric procedures being offered, but they all share the same basic principle: They reduce stomach size (to about the size of your thumb), and bypass some of the intestine. The result is that people eat less—remarkably less—and don't absorb as much of what they eat. The same can be accomplished by suturing the lips shut with just enough room for a swizzle stick. But you'd be hard pressed to find any surgeon willing to go along with that.

The rate of complications with this surgery is somewhat higher than other surgeries, mainly because the people that need this kind of surgery are at a higher risk of surgical complications because of their weight. Ironic, isn't it?

There are prescription pills available for those who are so inclined. Unfortunately, they are not the magical cure we hoped they would be. At best, they'll take off ten to twenty pounds, and only in conjunction with diet and exercise.

The over-the-counter supplements fare even worse. Regardless of what the bottle says, regardless of how much they'll 'boost metabolism', regardless of how much fat they'll 'melt away', they are even less effective than the prescription pills. It's the modern version of the old 'snake oil' sellers who rolled into town on their wagon touting the vitalizing and strength-giving properties of their products. By the time the townsfolk realized they'd been had, the wagon had moved on to the next locality. And almost all of these supplements have the fine print caveat that they only work when used in conjunction with a structured weight-loss program. If that's the case, taking a breath mint a day will help someone lose weight *and* freshen breath at the same time. We could call them 'thin mints' if it weren't for those darned Girl Scouts! (Flash Exposé: Girl Scout cookies are *not* made by Girl Scouts. It's true! And to think of all the years I spent admiring their packaging skills! But I digress.)

What this all boils down to is the same thing we've suspected, but hated to admit, all along. The best way to lose weight is to reduce caloric intake and increase caloric output.

But before you tear out this page, trample it, and burn it in frustration while doing a war dance with your face painted, keep in mind that 'dieting' doesn't have to mean 'eating corrugated cardboard three times a day'. (Eating it twice a day should suffice, being sure to take it with plenty of water.) Short of that, simple portion control can also make a huge difference. You can continue to eat the foods you like, but less of them. The CDC web site, *www.cdc.gov*, has a great section under 'obesity' called 'portion distortion' which gives great examples of how portion sizes and, as a result, obesity, have increased over the last twenty years. Portion control isn't as flashy or rapid as surgery or Atkins, but it is certainly more sustainable and less risky.

Gangster Hair Loss

Pop quiz, readers! What medical condition has the most late-night television commercials and its own club? No, there is no erectile dysfunction club . . . that I know of. Guess again. OK, obesity does, but that's not what I was going for. Look at the title. That's right—hair loss!

The medical term for hair loss is alopecia, pronounced al-o-PEE-shee-uh (although, to me, it sounds more like a gangster film actor than a medical condition—as in 'starring Al O. Pecia in 'The Receding Fella').

Just as there are many types of gangster films (mafia, hip-hop, and rehabilitated), there are many types of alopecia. Alopecia can be caused by medical treatments such as chemotherapy, by infections like fungi, or by medical conditions such as low thyroid. But the most common type is androgenic alopecia aka 'male pattern baldness.' It is characterized by hair loss on the top of the head. As the name suggests, it afflicts mostly men (up to two-thirds of men) but can, on rare occasions, affect women.

Male pattern baldness is so common that it's actually considered a 'normal variant' rather than an actual disease. And yet, few other 'normal variants' cause such distress in patients.

The culprit in male pattern baldness is testosterone which, ironically, is the same hormone that promotes hair growth on the rest of the body. While this may look like a recycling program, it's not.

In people who are susceptible to male pattern baldness, testosterone makes the hair follicles an offer they can't refuse. Most of the follicles, perhaps for fear of the family pet's safety, stop making hair altogether. Those that dare continue make short, fine hair—perhaps as an attempt to go undetected by testosterone's lackeys.

One can use this knowledge to gauge the historical accuracy of one's favorite gladiator movies. If the eunuchs in said movies are sporting full heads of hair, then at least the eunichs are depicted accurately. (Since eunuchs make no testosterone, they do not undergo male pattern baldness.)

But nowadays we have better treatments than that.

A Google search for male pattern baldness treatment yields 236,000 results. Given that there are only three treatments available, that should come out to 78,666 hits each. Surprisingly, it does not. Therefore, it would be wise to exercise caution when exploring one's treatment options. If the treatment in question is anything besides finasteride (Propecia), minoxidil (Rogaine), or hair transplantation, then there is no evidence that it works.

Finasteride and minoxidil are medications that block the effect of testosterone on the hair follicles. This means that they will prevent further hair loss. Some people might have some hair regrowth, but the main effect of these medications is to maintain follicular status quo.

Finasteride is a pill that is taken once a day, while minoxidil is a shampoo that is applied twice daily. They both stop hair loss rather quickly, but regrowth of hair can take up to two years.

Hair transplantation is a surgical procedure where hair from other parts of the head/body is taken and placed on the top of the head. It's invasive, but has a fairly good success rate. It is a very effective treatment for people who want to see a more immediate increase in their hair density.

Since male pattern baldness isn't technically a disease, getting insurance companies to pay for treatment is like asking the Godfather for a loan forgiveness program.

So to all those men, and few women, who are troubled by the larger clumps of hair in the sink and the receding hairline, be not afraid. Help is available without having to owe a 'favor'. The sooner it is sought out, the better. Meanwhile, look for the new Al O. Pecia movie 'Transplant This!' coming this Thanksgiving to a theater near you.

Happy Father's Day, ED

I've been feeling very manly as of late. Everywhere I turn, there are ads for masculine things: power tools, barbecues, golf clubs and pinky rings, to name a few. Father's Day tends to bring that out in Corporate America. Being the obedient consumer that I am, I've been adopting a more masculine outlook as well. I stand squarely, shake hands firmly, and ask my friends if they saw 'the game' last night. 'Boy, that Kobe sure can swing a bat!'

As I look at the muscular, chisel-faced, khaki-wearing, hilltop-standing, perfect-teeth-smiling man staring back at me from the L.L. Bean catalog, I console myself by thinking that since I have more life experience, I must be more fun to be with! I also envision Catalog Man's greatest medical concern: Not prostate, not heart disease, but erectile dysfunction—the dreaded 'ED'.

Thanks to recent medications and the incessant direct-to-consumer advertising thereof (involving various sports personalities and movement of various sports equipment through other equipment), this handsome man might feel more comfortable talking to his doctor about his problem than his father or his father's father. (Or his uncle's UPS man . . . or his great-grandfather's grocer . . . or his cousin's stepfather's gardener. But I digress.)

We used to call erectile dysfunction 'impotence' which is a Greek term meaning 'without power.' But then it caused too much confusion during power outages: 'Did you hear the thunder last night? The whole block was impotent all night.' So the term 'erectile dysfunction' was coined in order to be more specific.

Erectile Dysfunction (ED) encompasses many things. It can mean difficulty with getting a full erection. It can mean an erection that doesn't last. It can mean difficulty with erections in certain situations. It can also mean the complete lack of erections.

When thinking about ED, the song 'Big Yellow Taxi' by Joni Mitchell comes to mind. In it she sings, 'Don't it always seem to go, that you don't know what

113

you've got 'til it's gone . . . '. Most men don't fret over their erectile abilities until they start to dysfunction.

All evidence and anecdotal experience to the contrary, an erection is a rather complicated process. The correct floodgates have to open and close at the right time and for the right *length* of time to allow blood to flow into, and stay in, the designated area. It involves nerves, arteries, veins, smooth muscles, and cartilage all working together to make it happen. If any of those elements are not functioning properly, ED pays a visit.

Until recently, the treatment for ED wasn't exactly user-friendly. There were injections into the area (ouch!). There was the complicated vacuum-and-ring method. (And we're not talking about the type a mother would buy from a traveling salesman. Or are we . . . ?) And there were implants, both permanent and inflatable. Not exactly the makings of a romantic evening.

Then came the 'little blue pill'. Originally designed as a drug to treat heart disease, it was a complete failure—or was it? Sure, it didn't keep the heart any healthier, but the men in the experiment were much happier. And who are we to say that it didn't, in some way, help to keep their hearts healthier as well?

Not to be outdone, other pharmaceutical companies soon put out their own 'me, too' versions of the drug. Suddenly, treating ED was as easy as having an after-dinner mint. Today, we have three to choose from: Viagra, Levitra and Cialis.

All three do the same thing: increase blood flow. All three are ready to do their duty within thirty minutes of ingestion. And during the drugs' active timeframe (four hours for Viagra and Levitra, and thirty-six hours for Cialis), in the right setting, they can make an evening memorable.

What these medications don't do, however, is increase one's desire for intercourse. In fact, the FDA recently gave a slap to the wrist of the manufacturer of one of these drugs because their ads implied that the drug helped increase desire. The manufacturer had to say it was sorry, stay after school, and write on the chalkboard 'I won't deceive consumers' one hundred times.

So Happy Father's Day, fathers! Here's hoping ED leaves us alone until all we care about is sitting in our rocking chairs telling the neighborhood kids to stay off our lawn. But if it should happen to seek us out sooner, we have new weapons with which to wage battle against this deadly disease. Long live failed experiments!

Have You Seen This Virus?

The Oscars and Emmys might be far away, but there is another, equally glamorous award that has already taken place. Each year, the Academy of Motion Picture Center for Disease Control and Prevention and Sciences, names the three strains of the flu virus that will be included in that year's vaccine.

It is a very tough competition. Hundreds, if not thousands, of strains of the flu virus all over the world compete for the honored distinction of being part of the vaccine. The CDC tracks the activity of different flu strains worldwide and picks the three it finds most promising. Then, at a star-studded, gala event, they reveal the winners. Even though there's only one category, the award show still runs over three hours thanks to the musical numbers, nostalgic pieces and two-and-a-half hours of commercials.

A 'strain' is the viral equivalent of a 'clone'. If all the members of the Screen Actors Guild (SAG) were flu viruses, then each individual actor would be a 'strain'. Each actor would also have millions of clones of him or herself. The CDC would watch box office records very closely to see which three actors have been the most active, and for, say, one particular year, they would most likely pick Alec Baldwin, Steve Carell, and Cate Blanchet. (Mr. Baldwin and Mr. Carell would get extra credit for doing regular television work.)

Since the flu vaccine is a 'killed' vaccine, there would be no Alec Baldwins in the syringe. Instead, there would be photos, video clips, clothing samples and possibly a tuft of hair: all the things one would need to recognize Alec Baldwin if one had never met him.

The body's immune cells then take the Alec Baldwin bits and study them thoroughly. Then they keep a vigilant eye out for Mr. Baldwin. If you think the Patriot Act is tough, the body's immune cells will destroy anything that is remotely foreign. They don't even ask questions later.

Much in the same way that photos and hair samples cannot star in a movie, the flu vaccine cannot cause the flu. Some people may have a slight fever or body aches, but that's just the immune system reacting to the vaccine. Also, the flu vaccine does not protect against the common cold, so it's possible to get a cold around the same time someone receives the flu vaccine. This would be a correlation and not causation. (For more details on correlation and causation, see chapter herein.)

Some astute readers may wonder what happens if the CDC gets it wrong and a strain different than the ones in the vaccine becomes the prevalent flu virus of the season. Luckily for us, the various strains of the flu virus have enough in common for the immune system to still recognize them. In other words, if Stephen or William Baldwin tried to enter the body, the immune system would still consider them foreign and deal with them accordingly.

Vaccine features aside, the other exciting part of the flu season is finding out if there will be enough vaccine to go around. Each year Americans await the news with baited breath like ancient Greeks outside the Oracle of Delphi. Will there be enough, or will we have to send our supplies by armored transport again? As it turns out, this year we have plenty of flu vaccine for everyone. While this certainly reduces the bragability of getting the vaccine, it is still good news for all.

So contact your healthcare provider to find out when the flu vaccine will be available. The sooner one is vaccinated, the better. Not only will it prevent a lot of discomfort and potential complications, it will keep those around you healthy as well by eliminating a potential source of transmission. As for Mr. Baldwin, Mr. Carell, and Ms. Blanchet, don't worry. If anything happens to them, I'm sure their clones will continue in their glorious footsteps. In fact, considering how busy they've been, I wonder if they have already put their clones to work! I'll have to ask them for the recipe.

A Head in the Game

One thing I've learned in my years in Carpinteria is that Carpinterians love football. The fact that this kind of football rarely involves the foot making contact with the ball doesn't seem to bother the throngs of fans that pack into Warrior Stadium on a Friday night to watch the Warriors compete.

For those of you unfamiliar with the game (and thus shunned from mainstream Carpinteria society), this kind of football is where the athletes get dressed in tight-fitting pants, large shoulder pads and helmets, and line up facing each other. Some are so friendly with the other team that they crouch down, get face to face and exchange pleasantries. The ball is then moved back to another player who gives or throws it to a third player, unless he can't, in which case he can wait or go forward and he still has the option to give the ball to another player, unless he has crossed the line that his team was lined up on initially. Meanwhile, all around him, other players are moving forward, unless they're moving back, being chased, or blocked, but not held—which is illegal. The play ends when someone with the ball falls down, or if the ball is dropped by a player, unless it didn't make it to the target and hits the ground. Points are scored by moving the ball into the zone at the end of the field, aka the 'end zone', or by kicking it through upright poles, unless the ball is drop-kicked in which case all bets are off.

It's really quite simple.

Amidst all the hustle and bustle, people bump each other and sometimes they get bumped in the head. If the bump in the head is strong enough, it can cause a 'concussion'. A 'concussion' is a bruise to the brain. The same way that a bruised muscle won't work properly, a bruised brain will temporarily have difficulty functioning as well.

Let's look at it from the brain's perspective: The little alien is sitting at the controls, watching through the giant double windshields that are our eyes. He is pulling levers, turning knobs and monitoring gauges and warning lights.

Suddenly, there's a strong impact that sends the little alien flying across the control room. He bangs his head on the back wall and gets a concussion himself. (How's that for irony?)

Meanwhile, the red overhead emergency light starts flashing; warning lights turn on all over the console; and a pleasant female voice lists in a very calm manner all the malfunctioning systems. The alien scrambles back to his Captain Kirk Collector's Edition Control Seat and starts flicking switches and pushing buttons frantically.

The balance centers are off. The sprinkler system in the memory room has turned on, soaking all new incoming information rendering it unusable. The stomach is feeling nauseous and the visual input centers are scrambling incoming signals, making them blurry. The concussed athlete feels dizzy, nauseous, and confused. He may have a headache and/or blurry vision. This is a grade one or 'mild' concussion.

If the blow is hard enough, the entire system shuts down. This is seen as a loss of consciousness. The little alien has to hit the restart button and wait for the system to boot up again. Sometimes it restarts right away. Other times it takes multiple efforts, including a call by candlelight to technical support and manually rewiring the system to get it to start again. If the alien gets the system restarted within two minutes, then it's considered a grade two or 'moderate' concussion. If it takes longer than two minutes, it's considered to be a grade three or 'severe' concussion.

Like any bruised body part, it's important to give the brain enough time to recover. Returning to activity too soon and getting a second concussion could result in severe brain damage. Coaches and athletic trainers evaluate athletes to see when they can return to activity.

An athlete with a grade one concussion who has been symptom free for fifteen minutes can return to the game that day. An athlete with a grade two concussion should be symptom free for one week before returning to activity. An athlete with a grade three concussion is done for the season, but may return next season depending on his progress.

So go Warriors! Advance the ball and score points! And watch those tackles with the head. If not for your sake, then for the little alien's sake.

HEADDSS Up, Teens

That smell of fresh stationery in the air can mean only one thing: Back to School! Or in my case, Sports Physical Season! This is that special time of year when teenagers come in to get physicals. It's a time for them to tell us everything is 'fine' and a golden opportunity for us to sneak in some intervention.

Almost always, the exam is normal and the teen can participate with no restrictions. But the big intervention is the HEADDSS assessment. The HEADDSS assessment is an acronym physicians came up with to help them remember all the things that need to be addressed with a teen. It stands for Home, Education, Activities, Drugs, Depression, Suicide, and Sex. (It replaced the less popular TTAILS assessment which stood for Totally Teasing, Awesomeness, I'm so sure, Lameness, and Stuff.)

'Home' means a teen's living situation. We ask how many humans and animals live at home—specifically what kind of humans (parents, siblings, etc.) and what kind of animals, since certain animals can carry certain diseases. We ask if there are any smokers or guns in the house. If so, we ask if they're locked away, unloaded, with the ammunition locked separately—the guns, that is. It's advised that the smokers quit or smoke outside every time wearing a smoking jacket (meaning a jacket that is worn while smoking—not one that is on fire.)

'Education' has to do with schooling: what grade are they in and how are they doing in school. It's worthwhile to know about relationships with peers and boyfriends/girlfriends. Asking about bullying (both giving and receiving) is a recent addition to this category due to its wide prevalence and underestimation. (The 'B' hasn't officially been incorporated into the acronym because 'HEBADDSS' sounds like a hip-hop artist.)

'Activities' is everything else the teenager does outside of school. Popular items include sports (especially with teens getting a 'sports physical'), music (playing and listening), and the ever-popular 'hanging out with friends'. It's always reassuring to hear a teenager engage in these normal adolescent behaviors.

'Drugs' specifically refers to the illegal kinds. If so, we ask what kind, how often, and give strong advice to quit.

Depression is common amongst adolescents. Virtually all teenagers have moody spells (up to twenty-five hours per day), but the task is to differentiate normal teenage moodiness from true depression. If a teenager withdraws from family, friends and things that they enjoy doing, or if their school performance worsens for no apparent reason, it could be a sign of depression.

Questions about suicide then follow. Teenagers are at risk for suicide and asking openly about it is a great opportunity for some meaningful intervention.

Sex (and by extension teenage pregnancy) is another big health risk. If a teenager is sexually active, it is helpful to know how many sexual partners they've had in their lives, if those partners were female, male, or both, and if they have used anything to protect themselves from diseases and pregnancy. A discussion about being tested for sexually transmitted diseases (STDs) usually follows.

But perhaps the biggest irony of the sports physical is that these teenagers are the ones least likely to need any intervention. Teenagers who participate in sports have a lower likelihood of using illegal drugs or having sex.

The teenagers who are most at risk for using drugs and having sex are the ones who don't do sports and thus don't come in at all. But, with the adolescent visit, every encounter is a golden opportunity not to be missed.

On the parents' side, discussing alcohol, smoking, drugs, and sex can make a big difference in a teenager's behavior. Of course they will roll their eyes and groan, 'Moooommmm' or 'Daaaaaddd', but I believe that deep down inside, they're grateful for the concern. They just can't show it because it's against the rules.

So good luck to all athletes this coming school year. Good luck to all parents in getting through another year of middle school or high school. And even if your teen does not engage in school sports, do consider having him/her get a physical each year. It can make a big difference in their present and future health.

Healthonomics

The current economic state has been called many things: a downturn, a recession, a crisis. Personally, I make it a point to shamelessly compliment any entity that is about to come into a large sum of money. So to the economy, I say, 'My, how global you've become!' And 'Your interest rate looks lower. Have you been working out?' At this point, I would casually touch the economy in a non-threatening way on the elbow, while subtly mimicking its body language. The next thing I know, the economy will be off flirting with some public works company leaving me to wonder if I'd overdone it with the aftershave.

But whilst the nation awaits with baited breath to see if the various stimulus packages will work, many people are having to face the possibility, or the reality, of losing their jobs. As if losing one's income and livelihood were not enough, in the American healthcare system, losing one's job also means losing one's healthcare coverage—arguably when it is needed most.

Once healthcare coverage is lost, for the healthy person, it becomes imperative to keep from getting ill. For people with chronic illnesses, it becomes a matter of controlling those illnesses as well as possible. To that end, here are some tips that can help.

Sleep: Besides helping with obtaining and maintaining a healthy weight, getting adequate sleep has been shown to boost the immune system. A boosted immune system can fight off colds and the flu more readily. Most people need seven to eight hours of sleep each night to reap this benefit. (I have now mentioned sleep in several chapters. Tune in to my next book when I'll be writing about sleep's ability to fight terrorism!)

Staying active: Becoming and staying active has also been shown to boost the immune system and help just about any chronic illness known to man, woman, child, or pet (with the possible exception of 'the mange'). Doing an activity that one finds enjoyable and making said activity a part of the regular routine both help to maintain a more active lifestyle. Being active also improves sleep quality. To complete the cycle, being rested helps with alertness and motivation during the day to maintain an active lifestyle. It's like a 'healthy living' shampoo: lather on the exercise, rinse away with sleep, repeat.

Eating well: Eating good foods in good amounts can keep the body healthier as well. An economic recession/crisis/downturn is a strong incentive to eat out less often, which is a very good start. Eating more meals at home, in and of itself, is a healthier way to eat. The other part to address is the composition of said meals. Foods made with vegetables, beans, and legumes can help with many chronic illnesses including diabetes, high blood pressure and cholesterol. Limiting starches and meats can give an additional boost to the health-giving properties of a home-cooked meal. For you altruists out there, eating less animal products is also a great way to fight green house gasses. Apparently, livestock are prolific gas factories. I salute the brave scientists who decided to conduct those experiments and hope that none of them smoked on the job.

The best part is that all of these habits can also help in coping with the stress of having to find work or trying to keep a job. Being mentally and physically healthier allows one to do his/her job better or to make his/her job search more effective.

So as we all brave this storm together, let's eat well, get/stay active, and get enough rest. Soon this will all be a tale we tell our or other people's grandchildren about 'the old days' as we shake our heads at their extravagant lifestyles and blatant disregard for their elders' sage advice. And what is it with that hair?

Health Reform Part 1

It's been awhile since the *Patient Protection and Affordable Care Act,* aka health reform, became law. The law was not named *American Longevity and Affordable Care Act* because that would spell ALPACA and if health reform were to be a beast of burden, it would have to be an American one. Legislatures had difficulty reaching a concensus on a good acronym. Democrats proposed *Don't Overcharge Now, Keep Everyone Yearning* aka DONKEY, but that did not make a lot of sense. Republicans proposed *My Useless Lame Excuse,* aka MULE, but that was deemed too bitter. (Both parties wisely stayed away from *American Salubriousness Services*).

Nevertheless, health reform has passed and all that remains now is to enforce it or repeal it, depending on one's political leanings. But for a piece of legislation that ignited such fierce debate and invoked images of utopia and armageddon, it sure is going to take its sweet time. Some measures will go into effect this year, but the big ticket items, like insurance exchange pools, and free coverage of preventative services won't be enacted for a few years to come. I believe The Gap has the same idea when it places sale items in the back of the store.

Full details of the plan are beyond the scope of this chapter. However, here are some highlights as to what we can expect this year. The information in this chapter was researched from the following websites: *dpc.senate.gov,* which is the senate's own website and has a summary of the bill, the Kaiser Family Foundation *www.kff.org,* and *www.cnn.com.* Research was also done on *www.eightminutepecs.com,* but not for this article.

Starting this year, children will be able to stay on their parents' health insurance until they're twenty-six years of age. Unfortunately, there is no requirement for them to have to move out of the house to be eligible. (Although, if the child is not aware of that, the parent is not obliged to divulge.)

Another reform for 2010 is that health insurance companies will have to justify increases in premiums to the Health and Human Services (HHS) Secretary. And it had better be good! Claiming they lost their wallet that had all the money to provide health insurance to their clients will no longer cut it. They will now have to file a police report and submit a copy to the HHS Secretary. The HHS Secretary, in turn, reserves the right to give them all the suspicious looks he/she can over his/her reading glasses.

Also in 2010, health insurance companies will no longer be able to exclude children with pre-existing conditions. So all those children with stubbed toes can finally get the coverage they deserve. And while some might still be excluded from schoolyard games due to cooties, at least their parents will be able to indicate that on their insurance application without fear of being denied coverage.

Along the same lines, insurance companies will no longer be able to drop people who become ill. (Unless one is on fire, in which case they must first be stopped and then rolled after dropping.) No clearance is needed from the HHS Secretary.

And that's just the beginning! There is much more health reform to be implemented this year. Tune in to the next chapter for more on what to look forward to or dread. There won't be any big ticket items on that list, either, but so long as we all keep our expectations low, it could be just as titillating. Especially now that we can all titillate with reckless abandon since it won't jeopardize our healthcare coverage.

Health Reform Part 2:
Just Wait and See

Health reform is still relatively young. If it were a normal baby, it would be smiling spontaneously, cooing, and having about six wet diapers a day. That's about the extent of health reform's activities thus far. But it still has potential.

Previously, we covered some of the changes to expect this year. In this chapter, we continue our journey down the pot-holed road of health reforms for 2010, staying directly down the center of the lane to avoid the rotten fruit being tossed from the right and the rose petals being thrown from the left.

Starting within ninety days of the law passing, a new high risk pool was formed to cover patients who have pre-existing conditions and cannot get health insurance on their own. One can think of it as a social networking site where people who can't get health insurance coverage meet and exercise their collective bargaining power to buy health insurance. And, OMG, the government will help subsidize the group!

Also this year, all the senior citizens who fell into the 'donut hole' of Medicare part D will receive a check for $250. In order to fall into the 'donut hole', one's medication expenses must exceed $2400 for the year, or over $200 per month. So this rescue check will provide a month's worth of medications. In other words, all the senior citizens in donut holes across the country will have a one-rung ladder sent their way. If their donut hole is only one rung deep, they're in good shape. If it's any deeper than that, at least they can be one step closer to the fresh air at the top of the well whilst they await the great crane of January 1st to pull them out.

But of all the reforms that will take place in 2010, these last two are the most intriguing to me. One is the establishment of non-profit Patient Centered Comparative Effectiveness Outcome Research Institutes. (Perhaps next year we could reform their names to something shorter.) Basically, these are institutes who compare different treatments to see which is better. While this may seem like common sense, this type of information is actually very hard to come by.

For a new drug to be approved, it only has to work better than a placebo, aka nothing. But the question of whether it's better than what's already in use remains unanswered. Comparative effectiveness research tries to answer those types of questions. One famous example was a study conducted by the National Institute of Health regarding blood pressure medications. They found that a cheap, generic, water pill was more effective than any of the newer, more expensive medications. Comparative effectiveness research can also be applied to new procedures, like virtual colonoscopies and digital mammography.

One caveat of the bill is that the results of comparative-effectiveness research may not be used by insurance companies to dictate how doctors treat patients.

The other very intriguing piece of health reform for 2010 is that health insurance companies will be required to report how much of their revenue is spent on healthcare versus administration and overhead. If they spend less than 85 percent of their revenues on providing healthcare, they are to provide a refund to their clients. Perhaps we'll see a surge in healthcare spending by insurance companies when it's time to report their annual revenue with roving agents handing out free nicotine patches, pedometers, and blood pressure machines.

There are other reforms that will go into effect this year and reforms will continue to roll out until 2014 when there is expected to be a big graduation party for health reform, provided it does not drop out or get expelled for doing drugs which would be really ironic. For those interested in learning more about health reform, further details can be found at *www.healthreform.gov*, the government's website on health reform. For those not interested in health reform and looking for an effective treatment for insomnia, further details can be found at *www.healthreform.gov*.

Herpes 1 and Herpes 2

The spots had come out. The pain had begun.
Oh, how they burned. Something had to be done.
I went to my doctor. I said, 'Tell me true.'
What do I have? Herpes 1 or herpes 2?
The good doctor said, ' Tell me what you felt.
Was it above the neck, or below the belt?'

'Above the neck,' I said with chagrin.
'But not on my nose, and not on my chin.
Right here on my lips, these three spots, do you see?
What can I do? Oh, what could it be?'

He looked at my spots. They were small. They were red.
They had little fluid bubbles that formed a small head.
'This is herpes, type 1.' Then he gave me a pat.
'How do you know?' I said as I sat.

'Cause it's on your head, right there on your lips,
And not on your elbows and not on your hips.
You got these spots from someone before.
Someone, like you, who had lips that were sore.

When you touched the sores, the virus was there,
And besides saliva, that's what else you shared.
The virus got under your skin very quick.
It hid for a while, and now makes you sick.

But have no fear,' he said with a smile.
'I'll give you some medicine, they'll go in awhile.'

So he gave me the prescription, and I was so glad,
To be done with this painful infection I had.
I smiled at the pharmacist as she dished out the pills.
She said, 'Take five a day, for a week, if you will.'

It was called 'acyclovir.' I took the full course.
The spots were all gone. I was fit as a horse.
So I called up my girlfriend and told her the news.
I said, 'Don't be afraid, and don't get the blues.

Everything's gone, I'm fine, do you hear?'
She said, 'I know that you are, but there's something else, dear.'
For I have had spots and they have been sore.
I tried to wait but I can't any more.

So I saw my doctor and told her the story.
I told her everything and then some more-y.
She said I had herpes, it was number 2.
I have been tested and now so should you.'

'But how do I do that? Where do I go?'
'Go ask your doctor,' she said, 'he'll know.'
So I went there again. I said, 'Pardon, doc.
You gave me some medicine and the pain did stop.

But my girlfriend, she got them, but not where I thought.
Hers are below the belt, mine were up top.'
'Then she has herpes type 2,' the doc said.
'It is good that you came in. There's nothing to dread.

We can test you for herpes two. Yes, we can.'
He gave me an order, and to the lab I ran.
The next day he called me. The blood test confirmed.
I had herpes 2, that's what I had learned.

The doctor explained, 'You might get some spots,
Below the belt this time, they might hurt a lot.
Tingling and burning are signs of a flare.
Take the acyclovir. Take it with care.

These spots will come back. They usually do.
Pretty often the first year, and less in year two.
And with each year that passes by,
Fewer spots will meet your eye.'

And that's how I learned about the herpes disease.
There are two of them, type 1 and type 2, if you please.
Type 1 is on top, 'round the lips, to be sure.
Type 2 is below the belt, they both can recur.

So if you get spots that are red and they're sore,
Be it at home, or out in the store,
Go see your doctor and let him/her check.
Get tested and treated and don't go through heck.

The medicine helps, don't you forget'em.
But the best thing, of course, is try not to get them.
Know your partners and if they have spots,
Talk about it some, before things get hot.

Avoid contact with herpes spots, this part, don't omit.
And may you always stay happy, and healthy, and fit.

In honor of the late great Dr. Seuss who didn't write nearly enough medical text books.

Home, Sweet Medical Home

Words like 'universal coverage', 'portable' and 'Health Savings Accounts' are already quite in vogue these days. But there is a new term that we may start to hear, the 'medical home'. The idea of a 'medical home' was first proposed by the American Academy of Pediatrics (AAP) in 1967. They simply recommended that a child's medical records be archived in a single location. While that may sound like common sense now, apparently it wasn't so in 1967. They also wanted a dog and a white picket fence surrounding each chart but that was deemed unreasonable since white picket fences clash with Spanish-style architecture.

But then, in 2007, the American Academy of Family Physicians (AAFP) and the American College of Physicians (ACP) joined the AAP in giving the 'medical home' concept an extreme makeover. They envisioned what they would want in an ideal primary care office and put it down in writing like our forefathers did more than 200 years ago. They called it 'Patient-Centered Medical Home' (PC-MH).

The revised statement starts with the introduction, 'The Patient-Centered Medical Home is an approach to providing comprehensive primary care for children, youth and adults.' (I would have suggested, 'We, the Primary Care Providers of these United States of America . . . ', but that's just me.)

Under the PC-MH, each patient has a primary care provider who leads a team of individuals (i.e., nurses, reception staff, medical records, etc.) in taking care of a patient. The personal physician takes care of the entire patient for acute care, chronic management, screening and end-of-life care.

The PC-MH model also calls for coordinated care—meaning that specialists, subspecialists, hospitals, nursing homes, home health agencies, and a patient's family and community all work together. The model calls for care to be facilitated by electronic records and registries to ensure that patients get the appropriate care when they need it. (Team-building retreats and rope courses are not explicitly recommended.)

Sound good so far? Well, hang on to your 'medical hats', 'cause we're just getting started! Quality and safety are hallmarks of the model. (Hallmark will be coming out with Medical Home house-warming cards next year.) The physician would advocate for the patient and would use evidence-based medicine to guide their decisions. They would do periodic self-assessments to make sure they were providing a good medical home and would involve patient feedback in that assessment.

PC-MH also calls for 'enhanced access' via open scheduling (i.e., same-day appointments), expanded hours, and new communication options, like email and web-based scheduling.

The authors of the statement wisely conclude with a section on payment. They argue that payment for physicians and clinics that provide medical homes should reflect the higher level of service provided. They call for recognizing the value of patient-care efforts that physicians and clinic staff provide outside of face-to-face contact. To close up any loop-holes, they also stipulate that this should not reduce face-to-face compensation. (Try and get out of that one, insurance companies!)

The authors also want the clinics and physicians to be reimbursed part of the money saved from reduced hospitalizations under this model and to be appropriately compensated for achieving measurable quality improvements—such as annual eye checks for diabetics, cholesterol checks, and colonoscopies for appropriate patients, to name a few.

So the PC-MH is an ideal that we can strive for. It seems reasonable that it would accomplish the goal of reducing 'fragmentation' in healthcare. Perhaps we will see this PC-MH come into being—if not entirely, at least in part. Studies have suggested that patients who have a medical home tend to stay healthier, have better control of their chronic health problems and are more satisfied with their care. It's a win-win-win situation!

Hot Summer of Movies

Hollywood has gone too far. I'm OK with 'The Da Vinci Code' banners on my home page. I'm OK with the Superman logo bursting through a soda can. I'm even OK with children's books based on the movie 'Cars'.

But to actually bring about climatic change throughout the world is a bit much. I blame Al Gore. Perhaps he is still bitter about losing the election in 2000 and is looking to make a mark in some way; so he became involved with a movie about global warming. And what better way to get people to go see your movie about global warming than to crank up the thermostat on the planet! It's brilliant! People looking for refuge on a hot day can turn to cool movie theaters and with their curiosities already peaked about the hot weather, a movie on global warming sure would sound interesting. I don't know how he did it, but would you expect anything less from the ingenious, self-proclaimed 'father of the internet'?

Around here it's been like a sunny day in Seattle. We're simply not equipped to deal with it. Nobody has air-conditioning, so we've been using fans to blow the hot, humid air around (which at times only makes us hot and humid with messed up hair-dos).

So how is one to keep cool in such warm weather? Certainly drinking cool beverages can help. But beware of caffeine. Yes, that 'elixir of the gods', that turbo-charge for the brain, that mover of intestines, can actually make things worse by causing dehydration.

Caffeine works as a diuretic, meaning that it causes the body to lose fluid. So that double venti-frappaccino-mocha-latte-hazelnut-non-fat-whip-cream with a dash of cinnamon, while tasting very good at the moment, can act as a life-preserver made of lead—or an oxygen tank filled with carbon dioxide. It can actually wind up making things worse.

Caffeine can be sneaky. We all know it's in coffee. Most people know it's in soda. Some know it's in tea. Your best bet is to read the ingredients on any drink and see if it's there.

Another diuretic is alcohol. That ice cold beer sure may taste good after a day of yard work, but it too can make you more dehydrated.

Clear liquids are a good way to keep hydrated. A liquid is considered 'clear' if it is acquitted of all charges. As an alternative to reviewing its criminal record, you can put a piece of print on the other side of the glass. If you can read the print, the liquid is considered 'clear'. Examples are water, ginger ale, and certain sports drinks. Orange juice, tomato juice, and spinach-carrot cocktail would not be considered clear.

Enjoying these drinks cold can help keep the body cool.

Another way to keep the body cool is to make the skin wet. Our bodies naturally do that by sweating. What cools the body is the evaporation of fluid from the skin. So getting the skin wet and standing in front of a fan can help cool the body.

Also, going into air-conditioned buildings, i.e., department stores and movie theaters, can give the body a break from the heat.

All these things can help prevent heat stroke and heat exhaustion which are what happens when the body starts to lose the battle against heat. Most at risk are young children and the elderly.

Signs of heat stroke and heat exhaustion include body aches, tremors, confusion, heart racing, and lack of sweat. If any of these symptoms develop, it's important to get medical help right away.

So have your ice cold non-alcoholic, non-caffeinated clear liquid in the air-conditioned movie theater. Your body will thank you and so will the movie industry. Meanwhile, Al Gore gets the prize for best movie promotion.

Insight, So To Speak

One of the slogans of modern medicine could be, 'We never met an orifice we didn't probe.' Just like the Walt Disney Company did with sequels, the medical profession has systematically gone through all the orifices of the body and invented a way to look inside them. Some probings are not so bothersome, like the mouth and ears. But when you start going below the waist, things get a little uncomfortable.

When someone reaches the age of 50, they are a candidate for one of such probes. It's 'the scope'. People know it by many different names: colonoscopy, sigmoidoscopy, the giant snake-like thing, and the if-you-think-you're-getting-near-me-with-that-thing-you've-got-another-thing-coming.

The reason we go to these depths of the human body is for colon cancer screening. Just as there are many ways to skin a potato (as a cat owner, I can't get myself to say the other thing and considering that cat pelt has virtually no value, I'm not even sure how the saying got started), there are many ways to screen for colon cancer.

The most common screening method is a flexible sigmoidoscopy every five years combined with a stool test for blood every year. Notice the word *flexible* in 'flexible sigmoidoscopy'. That means that previously there used to be *rigid* sigmoidoscopies. As the name suggests, it did not bend. It was a straight hollow tube designed to be long enough to inspect the twelve-to eighteen-inch sigmoid colon. (The sigmoid colon is the very end part of the colon where most early cancers and polyps occur.) I had the misfortune of witnessing one during my medical school training at—where else—the VA hospital. And yes, it is exactly as uncomfortable as you imagine. The patient is positioned as if they're looking for something under a refrigerator and a lot of patience is exercised by patient and doctor. And like all VA patients, the patient in question joked all the way through the procedure and was very grateful afterwards. Hats off to all veterans everywhere!

Flexible sigmoidoscopy, by contrast, bends and twists to get around the sigmoid part of the colon. Relatively speaking, it's much more comfortable. Some places even have their scope connected to a television set so that the patient sees what the doctor sees. If you're uncomfortable watching your own insides on television, you can always pretend you're watching a spelunking special on the National Geographic Channel—*commercial free!*

A colonoscopy looks at the entire colon. It's a much longer tube, takes longer to do, and patients are generally sedated for the procedure.

The US Preventive Services Task Force (USPSTF) gives us these options for colon cancer screening after age 50: flexible sigmoidoscopy every five years, a stool test for blood that can't be seen with the naked eye every year, flexible sigmoidoscopy every five years *and* a stool test for blood every year, barium enema every five years and a stool test for blood every year, or a colonoscopy every ten years. (A barium enema is where liquid contrast is inserted instead of a scope and an X-ray is taken of the colon.) These procedures have all been found to be effective in catching colon cancer early. Treatment at the early stages of colon cancer tends to be more successful with fewer adverse effects.

What tends to direct choice is insurance coverage. Insurance companies have been much more willing to pay for a sigmoidoscopy every five years rather than a colonoscopy every ten years.

But in spite of all the gruesome descriptions and anecdotes, the part most patients find truly uncomfortable is 'the prep'. That's basically like the intense house cleaning people do before the in-laws come over. It involves drinking some special fluid that turns the colon into a high speed train track. It provides a good opportunity to catch up on a lot of reading—lots—and—lots—of—reading, in the privacy of your very own bathroom.

So be sure to keep your appointments for your yearly physicals—especially after age 50. You don't have to like the procedures, but bear in mind that for most people, it beats the alternative. At least these days you don't have to specify that you want the *flexible* scope.

Investigating Cold and Flu Supplements

If I were an investigative journalist, I would have professionals do my hair and makeup and I would have pictures of me with a serious expression plastered all over town. I would drive a fancier car (because I'd have an image to keep up), and dress in a casual, street-smart, yet accessible manner. One of my targets of investigation would be the alternative cold and flu remedy industry.

Alternative medicine is a bazillion-dollar-a-year industry—give or take a bazillion. Yet, there is scant proof of their efficacy.

As the well-known, cutting-edge, trim-haired, clean-shaven (except when out in 'the field') investigative journalist that I'd be, I'd drag my cameraperson out of bed bright and early one day and come knocking on the alternative medicine's door. I would start with one brand that seems to be particularly popular—the one that has the cartoon of a person with a large nose looking apprehensively at menacing 'bugs' floating about him on an airplane on the box. Let's call it 'Airhorne' for the sake of this discussion.

I would start with a direct, blunt question, getting right to the point. 'Is there any evidence of your product's efficacy in controlled, randomized trials?' When he slams the door in my face, I would run around the house, peek in a side window, and shout 'How is your product supposed to work?' When he runs and hides out of view, I would get the megaphone out and address him down the chimney, 'When was the last time you called a chimney sweep?'

Then, I would hide out somewhere in front of his house. When Mr. 'Airhorne' came out to go to work, I would charge ahead like George Washington crossing the Euphrates, shove a microphone in his face and ask, 'Your product claims to reduce the 'duration' of a cold. How do you define 'shorten'? Or 'duration' for that matter'

Having failed that, I would be forced to go undercover. I would disguise myself as a person with a cold by rubbing my face on a cat. I would go to Mr. Airhorne's place of business and ask for help. Then, I would ever so slyly slide in my questions:

'So, Mr. Airhorne, your product is supposed to 'boost' the immune system? How does it do that, exactly?' He would proceed to give me an answer that I would find clearly unsatisfactory.

'How did you determine that it 'boosts' the immune system? What kind of research was done? How did you measure the immune system's activity?' He would then provide me with a list of testimonials about people who have had success with his product. That's when I'd move in for the kill. 'But anecdotal evidence means nothing in clinical research. How do I know that for every one person with a success story there aren't 1,000 others who got no benefit at all? How do I know this isn't just a placebo effect?'

Then, I'd bait him. 'How did you get the FDA's approval for this supplement?' He would then inform me that since it's marketed as a supplement, it doesn't need the FDA's approval.

'In other words, you don't have to provide any proof for the claims you've made.' At this point, his highly muscular, well-dressed, and surprisingly polite security officers would show me the door—most likely head first.

That's when I'd cut back to the studio with me and the rest of the news team. I would give a look of indignation and recap, 'So, we basically found no evidence that this product does what it claims to do. There is no good research to support it.' The head newsperson would thank me for the interesting and thought-provoking report and say, 'Will the cold snap continue? Wiley Willie's Weekend Weather is next.'

I would do all that if I were an investigative journalist. But alas, I am not. So I guess I'll just stick to my writing.

IOU an IUD

Valentine's Day passed us by once again and the impact on the flower, greeting card, and K-I-S-S-I-N-G industry is astounding. But as we all learned in grade school, K-I-S-S-I-N-G leads to love, then marriage, and finally a baby in a jogging stroller so that mommy and daddy can regain their pre-baby fitness.

But with modern medicine, the baby part need not be an inevitable consequence of love and/or marriage. There are many ways to prevent unwanted pregnancies. One of the myriad of contraceptive choices available is the Intra-Uterine Device (IUD). 'Intra' means inside, 'Uterine' means uterus, and 'Device' means thingy. The name was created by the Marketing Group, Inc. marketing group.

The IUD is a small T-shaped device that goes inside the uterus. It is barely larger than an adult's thumb. As such, if one were to buy it in a dark alleyway, it could be easily transferred from person to person via a casual handshake. I imagine the exchange would go something like this:

'Do you have the device?'

'Yes. Do you have the money?'

'No. Bill my insurance.'

'What's your ID number?'

'I don't have that. '

'OK. How about your mother's maiden name?'

'I don't have that either.'

'How about your first pet's name?'

'I don't recall.'

'How about your first pet's maiden name?'

'Sorry.'

'Look, I can't help you unless you have an ID number . . . .'

But I digress.

Some people out there may have some rather unfond memories of IUDs. When the IUD first came out in the 70s, it wasn't exactly user-friendly. Some women experienced severe cramping and infections in the uterus. But then again, in those days, 'Pong' was on the cutting edge of home entertainment.

But much like the Wii system today makes 'Pong' look like a two-dimensional game with a square ball, modern IUDs make the old ones look like infectious cramp machines. The cramping with modern IUDs is much less and there is very little increased risk of infection.

So how does the IUD work? Once the IUD is placed inside the uterus, two things happen: One is that it invokes an anti-sperm attitude in the uterus. When sperm enter, they are forced down to the ground with their hands over their heads while something heavy sits on them indefinitely.

The second is that it makes the lining of the uterus inhospitable to a fertilized egg. So if a sperm were to find the egg, there would be no place for the egg to land. It would be like trying to find a spot for a new tattoo on Angelina Jolie's back. (Or so I've heard.) If the egg does not stick to the wall of the uterus, a pregnancy won't happen.

The ideal candidate for an IUD is a woman (obviously) who has had at least one child (the inside of the uterus is larger in women who have had children and thus the IUD is less likely to cause trouble) who has never had a sexually transmitted disease and is in a mutually monogamous relationship.

Of all these criteria, the last one is the deal breaker. The others would warrant a consultation with a healthcare provider.

Once inserted, the IUD can stay in for five to ten years, depending on the type used. It is very low maintenance, and thus has an effectiveness rate of 98 to 99.2 percent.

So to all the lovers out there K-I-S-S-I-N-G, whether in a tree or on the ground, you may not be able to choose when love comes. You may have some choice as to when marriage comes. But you certainly have a lot of choices when it comes to babies in carriages and when looking at said choices, consider giving the IUD a spot on the list.

Is a Shot, Is Not a Shot

My heart goes out to all pre-kindergartners who are coming in for their pre-kindergarten physicals. They are old enough to keep their panic at bay (up to a certain point) and smart enough to realize that going to the doctor's office when you're not sick can mean only one thing: shots!

The first and foremost thought on the minds of these four- and five-year-olds is, 'Am I going to get a shot?' Some are brave enough to ask the question as soon as they walk into the exam room. When we answer 'Yes', the next question is, 'How many?'

To me, a shot is a vaccine. A vaccine is given to prevent an illness. But to a pre-kindergartner, any sharp object piercing their skin is a shot. So after I explain that there are three shots, a finger poke to check for anemia and a tuberculosis skin test (which involves putting fluid under the skin with a needle), their eyes widen and they ask me incredulously, 'Five???' I nod my head sympathetically and add, rather sheepishly, 'But you get to pick out a toy afterwards.'

So even though the tuberculosis skin test is an injection using a needle, it does not prevent any illnesses. It is designed to see if the tuberculosis bacterium has ever been in the body. It's like in the old western movies where there's a lull in a shootout and the comic relief side-kick hiding behind a rock raises his hat to see if the assailants are still around and has a volley of bullets launched at his hat and when he brings it back down into the screen, there's pasta straining in it.

The tuberculosis skin test (aka PPD) works on the same principle, except instead of a hat, we use pieces of the tuberculosis bug and, instead of a volley of bullets, the injection site gets hard to the touch. This reaction only happens to people who have had the tuberculosis bug in their body at some point in their lives.

But the reaction doesn't occur until 48 to 72 hours after the fluid is placed. That is why a PPD test needs to be 'read' 48 to 72 hours after administration.

The 'reading' does not involve sitting in a dark room with incense, gazing into a crystal ball while drinking tea. That is not to say that it cannot be done in that manner; it's just not a requirement. Also, most malpractice insurance carriers frown upon such theatrics. (Speaking of which, anybody looking for a gypsy outfit? It's barely used.)

The 'reading' of a PPD involves a nurse or other provider feeling the injection site for hardness. If hardness is present, it is measured to see how big the area of hardness is and that gives the reading.

If someone has hardness of the correct size, then they, at some point, have come into contact with tuberculosis. That is all the test tells us. The next step is to determine whether the tuberculosis infection is present and active, present and dormant, or not present anymore—meaning that the body's immune system won the shoot-out and tuberculosis rode out of town.

But the timing of the read is crucial. If someone comes back before 48 hours or after 72 hours, the test is unreliable and has to be repeated. As anyone who has children knows, it's difficult to commit to dinner whilst seated at the table with the food in front of you—much less returning in 48 to 72 hours. So, unfortunately, some readings are missed and the kids wind up having to repeat the test.

So whether we call it a shot or not, the PPD test is still an important part of a well-child checkup. As for the kindergartners, they actually do quite well. As they're walking down the hall, tears drying on their little cheeks, toy and stickers in tow, most of them will turn and say 'Thank you.' I'm not sure what they're thanking me for, but I hope I'm that brave and forgiving the next time I need *my* PPD done.

Is it the Flu, or Is it the Flu?
(Respiratory vs. Intestinal Flu)

WARNING: Do not read this chapter before or while eating. Or immediately after. In fact, it's best read when you're hungry and trying to lose weight.

Lately I've heard harrowing tales from friends, family and patients about nights and days spent in the bathroom suffering the reversal of the usual alimentary flow, aka vomiting. They promptly proceed to describe in graphic detail consistency, color, and scent to which I respond, 'You had me at hello'. Some people think it's food poisoning, but most people call it the 'flu'. (Insert dramatic music here.)

Some of these hurlers have been those fortunate souls who knew—or slept with—the right people and received a flu vaccine this year. They lament that they still caught the flu despite the vaccination.

To these brave patrons of public health, I say, 'Fear not! For the real flu hath yet to come!' (This phrasing was brought to you by your local Renaissance Fair.)

When most people think of the 'flu', they picture the above scenario. However, the real 'flu', the one we usually have a vaccine for and the one that kills people, is the respiratory flu. Since it is a respiratory infection, the symptoms are restricted to the respiratory system. Since nobody breathes with their intestines, vomiting and diarrhea are not a part of it.

Let's take a journey. Imagine you're an air particle. Around here, you are likely in the shape of some type of pollen. You're happily drifting through the air and suddenly get sucked into a dark, humid space, with large tentacles, and howling winds. You have just entered the nose. Provided you don't get sneezed out, you then move on to a more spacious, less hairy, dark and moist place known as the throat. Then you whirl down a round tube, like the ones they have at water parks. This is called the trachea or the 'wind pipe'. (Not to be confused with bag-pipes.) You continue whizzing along, noting that the tube keeps getting smaller and smaller, until you're stuck in a tiny bubble.

This is the alveolus. It's the end of the line. You don't have to go home, but you can't stay here. This is where the lung does its business—oxygenation. Red blood cells cruise by dumping out waste and picking up precious, nourishing oxygen. This concludes your tour of the respiratory tract. Please watch your step on the way out and don't forget to stop by the gift shop.

So the respiratory flu will give you symptoms that are confined to the respiratory system: cough and sore throat. There is also intense body aches and high fevers (up to 104 degrees) at no extra charge.

Currently, flu activity in California is 'sporadic'. In fact, flu activity in the entire nation is 'low'. The CDC has a great map on its website, *www.cdc.gov*, showing flu activity in each state and it is updated weekly.

The intestinal 'flu' on the other hand, seems to be quite wide spread right now, as determined by my own thoroughly unscientific singular viewpoint. The typical course is vomiting for a day or two, followed by diarrhea for the next three to five days. The beauty of it is that, once you get it, there isn't a single thing any of us can do to make it go away. Fortunately, our body has figured it out. (I can't reveal all the details because I've been sworn to secrecy.) However, during the nausea phase, the BRAT diet helps. BRAT is *not* a reference to any of your younger siblings, but stands for Bananas, Rice, Applesauce and Toast. These are things most easily digested. Small, frequent amounts of fluid help keep the body hydrated. The diarrhea runs its course in about 3-7 days, which is a great opportunity to catch up on some reading. Always look on the bright side.

So the next time you run into someone with the 'flu', take a moment to clarify to which 'flu' they are referring. Is it the intestinal or the respiratory variety? You'll probably catch it anyway, but at least you'll have a heads up as to where you'll be spending your days: in bed or . . .

It's All in the Wrist

Our hands have been the subject of many proverbs, songs, and charity events. 'Hands Across America' attempted to form a human chain across the country to raise money to fight hunger and homelessness. There were many gaps in the chain but the organizers still stuck with 'Hands Across America' because the song was already recorded and 'Human Chain With Just a Few Gaps, Across Almost the Entire Nation' just didn't have the warm fuzzies.

Then there's the famous expression about idle hands doing the devil's work, such as shooting spit wads at unsuspecting angels and then quickly looking away.

But our hands would be unable to do any of these things without our wrists. Our wrists supply our hands with blood, nerves, and a physical attachment to the rest of the body. Quite a few of the muscles that move the hand are actually located in the forearm and control the fingers via tendons that run through the wrist—like really old-school telecommuters.

This makes the wrist a very crowded place, like a Tokyo subway train at rush hour. There is very little wiggle room. So if the index finger tendon doesn't like the way the ulnar artery is breathing on it, that's just too bad.

As late night infomercials have consistently shown us, using a muscle makes it bigger. (Apparently, even if it's just ten minutes a day, three days a week, as long as one can make three easy payments of $19.95.) Now let's suppose that one is part of a volunteer organization named after a famous blanket-loving Peanuts character that makes and donates home-made quilts and afghans to needy children all over the country. The repeated use of hand muscles in knitting and crocheting can make them bigger over time.

This becomes problematic because of the median nerve. The median nerve enters the hand right down the middle, at the base of the palm, between the two big muscles just below the thumb and the pinky.

Normally, these three structures are like three slender people in an airplane aisle. Each has half of an armrest and enough room to wiggle their toes and cross their legs, provided they're contortionists. With prolonged and repetitive fine movement, it becomes more like a slender person in the middle seat of an airplane full of Sumo wrestlers. Not only does the median nerve not get any elbow room, but he has to turn sideways just to breathe.

When nerves get squeezed, they have a hard time doing their job which is to supply feeling and allow movement. People experience this as numbness and weakness. In the case of the volunteer blanketmakers, or 'blanketeers', they feel this as numbness and weakness in the thumb and index finger which is made worse with knitting and crocheting.

This is commonly known as carpal tunnel syndrome. 'Carpal' refers to the wrist. 'Tunnel' refers to the narrow space between the two hand muscles that the median nerve has to squeeze through, aka the middle seat of the airplane aisle. And 'syndrome' is a medical term meaning a collection of symptoms because 'thingy' sounds unsophisticated.

Treatment of carpal tunnel syndrome involves taking the pressure off the nerve with braces, reducing the inflammation with anti-inflammatory medications like ibuprofen (Advil, Motrin), physical therapy, and generally de-stressing the nerve with B-complex vitamins. Cucumber facials and mud baths have not been shown to be effective, although they haven't been shown to be harmful either.

If these measures don't work, surgery can create more space for the median nerve so it can breathe easier. It's like transferring it to a center seat in business class on a plane full of professional football linesmen.

So to all the good people who are using their hands for worthy deeds, may your wrist's structures all get along and not encroach upon one another. But if they do, effective treatments are available which do not involve doing work for any diabolical entities, provided they're not disguised as loveable creatures in need.

Dedicated to the great people of Project Linus.
(For more information, go to *www.projectlinus.org*)

Keeping up with the Bones'

I think it's imperative that we add a national holiday to the month of August. Much like how Christmas sales start on November first, back-to-school sales start on July fifth. Therefore, if we had a commercially lucrative holiday in August, we could spare our poor children the angst of having to deal with back-to-school promotions when they still have a good six weeks of vacation left.

I propose we designate August 12 as American Co-Dependence Day. It would serve as a nice balance to all the Independence of July 4 and still give us enough time to have back-to-school sales. The greeting cards would read, 'I'll have a happy Co-Dependence Day if you do!'

But made-up August holidays or not, school is coming back like the swallows returning to San Luis Obispo. For many students, being back in school means resuming competitive sports. With sports come camaraderie, physical fitness, and the ever-present risk of injury, such as broken bones.

Our bones are the strongest structures in our body. That is why our muscles have chosen to attach themselves to them like a child clinging to the door frame to avoid going to the doctor for his/her broken bone. Since bones are so strong, it usually takes an extraordinary injury to break one. Most fractures occur below the elbow and below the knee. Maybe it's because these parts are more exposed. Maybe it's because they're further from the body and thus are more likely to wind up at an angle that can result in a fracture. Maybe it's because they look particularly good in a cast.

Whatever the reason, a broken bone is an injury that requires medical intervention. An X-ray is a helpful tool in determining if a bone is broken, aka fractured. When looking at an X-ray, doctors need to determine many things about the fracture, such as where the fracture is on the bone (i.e., the front, middle, or end), if it completely severs the bone, if the bone is still lined up correctly, and if there are multiple bone pieces at the fracture site, just to name a few.

The pain of a broken bone occurs partly from movement of the broken pieces. Therefore, a fracture on a weight-bearing bone, like the shin bone, hurts more because the pieces are more likely to move. A fracture on the fibula, the non-weight-bearing bone in the leg, might not be as painful since it doesn't move as much. Immobilizing the broken bone with a cast, splint, or pieces of wood bound by vines keeps the broken pieces from moving and can greatly reduce pain.

Painful as broken bones are, and as dramatic as the injuries that caused them can be, they are rarely life threatening as long as the bone isn't sticking out of the skin. Once it has been determined that a bone is broken, a 'splint' is applied, which can be a rather anti-climactic experience for the patient. After all that the injured person has been through, they wind up leaving the Urgent Care/Emergency Room with little more than a glorified bandage. This 'splint' usually has one or two hard sides and is wrapped with an ACE bandage.

The reason a flimsy-looking splint is applied at first instead of a robust cast is not because of time or budget constraints. It has to do with swelling. A broken bone reaches maximum swelling forty-eight hours after the injury. The soft sides of the splint allow the area to swell without cutting off circulation. After forty-eight hours, a regular cast can be placed and autograph requests may finally be granted.

So here's wishing all athletes a healthy and safe season. May you all enjoy the camaraderie, sportsmanship, and physical fitness of school sports. But if a bone should break, be assured that with the right treatment, it should heal just fine in four to six weeks. The hardest part will be the wait. In the meantime, it could be a good opportunity to plan the next Co-Dependence Day party—if your partner says it's OK.

Kindergarten Deconstructed

Dear 4- or 5-year-olds:

Are you searching for more in your life? Do you crave more interactions with your peers? Do you find the assignments at pre-school unchallenging? Do you want to take your mind and body to the next level?

Well, your search is over. Now there's *kindergarten*! Come and join the millions of children across the country who have taken this next step in their mental, physical, and social education. Just listen to these testimonials:

> *'I have fun.'*
> Tim, age 6.

> *'It's good.'*
> Elizabeth, age 5.

> *'I have a belly button.'*
> Abel, age 5 ½.

> *'I want a popsicle!'*
> Kim, age 6.

Sound too good to be true? It's not! You too can experience firsthand what it's like.

Kindergarten is a German word. *Kinder* means 'children'. *Garten* means 'Dear God, I need a break from these . . . '. It was started by ancient Germanic tribes who had the innovation to bestow the never-ending task of chasing after young children on hapless volunteers. Over time, these volunteers started to become professionals and soon were making almost as much as the poorest peasant in town (a tradition that continues to this day).

How do you sign up? It's simple. Your parents will take care of the application process. All you have to do is show up and be cute.

But kindergarten isn't for everybody. Side effects include, but are not limited to, making new friends, happier parents, learning new skills, and catching more colds. Consult your doctor to see if you are healthy enough to participate in kindergarten. Your doctor will examine you and then give your immune system a boost with usually three or four immune-boosting injections. After all, the entire purpose of school is defeated if you're home sick. Call now to avoid the late August rush!

But wait, there's more!

If you're among the first 65,528.36 people to come in for your kindergarten physical, we'll throw in height and weight measurements ABSOLUTELY FREE! See how you compare to your peers in size! See how much you've grown since you were two!

Space is limited and appointments are going fast. So start nagging your parents today to bring you in while you have time. Use the same approach you use to get them to take you to the beach—be it asking repetitively, or asking repetitively, or asking repetitively.

We look forward to seeing you at the clinic and keeping you healthy!

Sincerely,

Healthcare Providers of America

The Kissing Disease

I think St. Valentine should have been a little more considerate. While I appreciate having a romantic holiday in winter because the cold beckons physical closeness, I must question the wisdom of increasing demand for flowers at a time when only those with specialized facilities can grow them. I also don't think it's wise to flood restaurants with patrons on a night when it's uncomfortably cold to wait outside. Perhaps next year we can reconsider the date.

But humans are not the only organisms celebrating Valentine's Day. It's also a very joyous occasion for the Epstein-Barr virus, aka the causative agent of mononucleosis aka mono. (Incidentally, comedienne Roseanne Barr, and screenwriter Julius J. Epstein, who wrote the screenplay for 'Casablanca', were not involved in the discovery or naming of this virus—as far as I know.)

Mono is also known as the 'kissing disease.' Since the mono virus lives in saliva, kissing is a very efficient way of transmitting it. It's like door-to-door service in a heated vehicle with leather upholstery. But kissing is not the only way that mono gets around. Sharing utensils, cups and plates can also pass the virus around—although it's not as comfortable a transport for the virus as kissing.

Mono causes sore throat, swollen glands and fatigue. It tends to affect teenagers and young adults most. By adulthood, 95 percent of people have had mono which makes one wonder how the other 5 percent escaped it. Maybe they have enhanced senses that allow them to seek each other out in a sea of mono carriers.

The diagnosis of mono can be rather tricky since many other illnesses can cause a sore throat and swollen glands. To make it even more unfair, people with mono can have strep at the same time! There is a blood test available for mono, but it can be falsely negative early in the course of the illness. It's almost as if the mono virus is consciously trying to go undetected. I guess you don't get to infect 95 percent of the population if you go around advertising your presence.

Once the diagnosis of mono is made, most people begin to wonder from whom they got the illness. This can be a rather exhaustive search for some people since it can take thirty to sixty days for the symptoms of mono to show themselves.

The last great advance in the treatment of mono was the invention of rest. The first great advance occurred when liquid water formed on the earth. Anti-inflammatories, like ibuprofen, can help with the sore throat. The fatigue of mono can last for months.

But mono isn't just about kissing and resting. Nor does it only affect the throat and glands. Its most serious effect involves the spleen. The spleen is an organ that is located just under the ribs on the left side. Mono can cause the spleen to swell to the point that it sticks out below the ribs. Without the protection of the ribs, the spleen becomes more susceptible to injury. And when the spleen gets injured, it's a big deal. The spleen holds a lot of blood. If it gets injured, it can tear, causing people to lose large amounts of blood very quickly, which can be fatal.

Therefore, anyone with mono should avoid contact sports for at least four weeks after the onset of symptoms. For the teenage athlete, four weeks off sports is the equivalent of lifetime banishment on a deserted island without an iPod.

On the plus side, one can never get mono twice. This should not be taken as a kissing green light since there are plenty of other illnesses that can use the opportunity to infect a new host.

So for all the teens and young adults who have kissed and been kissed on Valentine's Day, set the clock. March 16 through April 15 is your target date. If you develop sore throat, swollen glands, and fatigue, it could be mono. If the symptoms start after April 15, then your Valentine's date is off the hook, provided the kissing did not continue beyond that date.

The Low-Down on Asian Bird Flu

It sucks to be a chicken in Vietnam right now. By chicken I mean the domesticated fowl, not the personality trait. By fowl I mean bird, not misconduct. Although I'm sure being a misconducting coward in Vietnam isn't any fun either.

The world is on full Bird Flu alert. Not since the great Alien Invasion of 1996, dramatically captured in the documentary film 'Independence Day', has there been such a united global effort against a common enemy. Jews and Muslims, Democrats and Republicans, and doctors and lawyers everywhere have set aside their differences and presented a united front. (We've chosen not to present our united backs because it's been really difficult to get to the gym lately with our hectic bird flu-containing efforts and all. But we do plan on going back. In fact, we just renewed our membership. These pants aren't exactly flattering, either. But I digress.)

The European manufacturer of Tamiflu, the human flu drug that *might* help with the Avian Flu has stopped shipment of the drug to the United States, because of concerns that we might 'hoard' the medication. To them I say, 'puhleeeeze!' Just because we have the highest obesity rate of any country and consume more energy than all of North Africa and parts of the Middle East combined, doesn't mean that we 'hoard' things. But I digress-or is it digest? I think they mean the same thing.

Why then, all the hype? Beside it being good news for people who love bad news which, according to popular media, is everybody?

The problem is potential. We already know that the Asian Bird Flu can infect humans. So far, it's only been people in direct contact with infected birds. There *may* have been a few cases of human-to-human transmission, but it hasn't spread beyond one person. The problem is that these flu viruses can mutate, acquiring abilities they didn't previously have. So if this virus becomes capable of spreading from human to human, the way regular human flu does, we'd be in big trouble. It could spread very quickly from person to person. We could have a pandemic, which is a global spread of a disease. The problem would be that our bodies aren't used to being infected by bird viruses and so are not very good at fighting them. The worst case scenario (which invariably gets more press coverage than the best case scenario) could result in millions of people dying in the US alone.

There are vaccines being developed. The situation is being monitored very closely worldwide. Lots of birds are being destroyed in order to contain it.

Some countries are drafting emergency plans involving limiting travel and large gatherings for weeks in case of an outbreak.

But as of now, none of this has happened. So what can we, as individuals, do to prepare? Fortunately, or unfortunately, not much. We can be assured that it will most likely take some time for any human-infecting strains of the bird flu to reach the United States. And, thanks to Hurricane Katrina, we've had a great chance to work out all the kinks in our emergency response system and so the good old US of A is the safest place to be, in my opinion.

On the plus side, this could be a chance to really use that emergency broadcast system that's been tested so much. I just hope that this time they make a clear distinction that it is *not* a test. The President jumping up and down on the TV screen yelling, 'THIS IS NOT A TEST, PEOPLE!' should suffice.

Also, let's keep in mind the best case scenario: that the flu will be contained and we'll have to pay a little more for Peking Duck in Tokyo.

Lumbago

Lumbago is not a tropical island with white sandy beaches, crystal clear waters, and all-inclusive resorts scattered along the edges of crushing urban poverty.

Lumbago is not the name of a bluegrass-zydeco fusion cover band.

Lumbago is not the new V8 350-horsepower Ford pick-up truck.

And yet, virtually everyone reading this has had first-hand experience with it. In fact, it is so common that The Kinks wrote the song 'Louie Louie' about it. Sing along: 'Louie, Louie. Ooooohhhhh baby. Lumbago . . . '

Lumbago is a catch-all term for back pain. In a recent survey of 1,543 adults, 120 percent of respondents reported having had back pain at some point in their lives. (The surveyors were subsequently forced to take remedial statistics.)

The human back is a marvel of biological engineering. Let's make one together: Just grab the nearest quadruped skeleton, swing it upright, tilt the pelvis back, curve the spine to accommodate, and hope for the best. Alternatively, take some blocks and stack them twenty-four high with Jell-O in between. It's like balancing a plate on a stick—but not as stable.

We've been walking upright for millions of years and still we're having trouble with our backs. The worst part is that no one can remember the customer support number. Heck, we didn't even save the receipt. Yet, were it not for our finicky backs, what would we do with all the shelf space now dedicated to acetaminophen (Tylenol) and ibuprofen (Advil, Motrin)? Back pain is a multi-billion dollar industry and employs thousands of people from cashiers to physical therapists to doctors and nurses. On the other hand, it costs billions of dollars every year in lost wages. So I suppose it all evens out.

Modern medicine, with all its might and fury, still hasn't cracked the case of back pain. (Pardon the pun only if you didn't think it was funny.) Our back is made up of vertebrae (the blocks), discs (the Jell-O), and layers upon layers of muscles, tendons, cartilage and ligaments. We have MRI machines that give us beautiful, crystal clear pictures of all the components of the human back. Yet when you compare most MRIs of people with back pain to those of people without back pain, there's hardly any difference.

So where's the pain? It's in there somewhere. Most of the time it tends to lie within those layers of muscles, tendons, ligaments, etc., but not in a way that can be visualized.

So what is one to do with an aching back? Tincture of Time (ToT). It is available virtually anywhere. (Prices may vary by location and occupation. Void where prohibited. Excludes tax and license. Not available in Nebraska.) The fact is that over 80 percent of back pain will go away in six weeks, in *spite* of any therapy. Muscular strains take about six weeks. Slipped or 'popped' discs take around forty-five days, and for pain from misalignment, expect improvement in about a month and a half.

Anti-inflammatories like ibuprofen can help. Beyond that, physical therapy, chiropractic treatments, and acupuncture have about the same effectiveness. It's not a bad idea to rest for the first day or two. Afterwards, you're better off being up and around walking. Keep in mind that the two positions least straining on the back are straight up and down, or lying flat. Any deviation stresses out your back muscles and they start being snooty.

So cheer up, you weekend warriors, you do-it-yourselfers, you I-just-reached-for-a-glass-of-water people! Relief is only six weeks away. Until then, curl up very straightly with a bottle of your favorite anti-inflammatory and boss people around.

DISCLAIMER: All this applies to acute back pain only—meaning back pain that is new. Chronic back pain is an entirely different bi-ped animal. Once back pain lasts beyond six weeks, it can legitimately be called chronic. The treatment then gets rather complicated. Since you asked nicely, I'll save it for a future chapter.

Magic Spray with a Side of RICE

I once heard the FIFA World Cup described as 'a foreign eccentricity that Americans tolerate every four years.' While that statement has become less and less true over the last few years, soccer is still far from the American every-day consciousness. If we were having a civil war, I'm not sure we would call it off to watch the US National Soccer Team play the Czech Republic. If we were oppressed and our civil liberties violated (hypothetically speaking, of course), I doubt we would use a victory/defeat by the US National Soccer Team as an excuse to stage new and re-invigorated demonstrations.

For those not familiar, the FIFA World Cup is a month-long soccer tournament where the top thirty-two teams in the world compete for the much-coveted trophy. As with any sport, injuries happen. The sequence is thus: a player goes down on the field, the referee goes over, checks the player, the referee faces the sideline and pantomimes carrying a breakfast-in-bed tray, the medics rush on the field, carry the hobbling player off, spray the affected area and, seconds later, the player is back on the field better than before.

The spray that soccer trainers use has come to be known as the 'magic spray'. What's it made of? I believe it's a delicate mixture of wing of bat, dragon morning breath, and pixie dust. I'm not sure if anyone really knows the true contents of the spray and frankly, it doesn't matter. Nothing works that quickly. Spraying an injured area is like telling a five-year-old to go looking for 'grunion' on the beach. It simply buys time.

When somebody is injured, let's say a 30-something weekend warrior who still thinks he's in his 20's and winds up hyper-extending his ankle while trying to tackle the ball away from a whale of an attacker with an incredibly life-like leg made of titanium alloy (again, purely hypothetical), there's damage to tendons and ligaments. The body's response is to try to heal the area via 'inflammation'. Inflammation causes swelling. So the treatment for a strain or sprain involves reducing inflammation and swelling.

This is done via RICE treatment. By RICE I don't mean that very special aromatic basmati that's grown in sub-tropical India by a family of left-handed rice growers who sow with the left hand but harvest with the right. No, RICE stands for Rest, Ice, Compression and Elevation.

Rest doesn't necessarily mean lying on the couch, buying magic sprays from late-night-basic-cable infomercials for three easy payments of only $19.95!! (Call now and receive a travel-sized magic spritzer absolutely free!!!) Relative rest also works. This means taking a break from heavy activity and doing lighter activity with the affected area.

Ice means placing ice or something cold on the affected area. Frozen peas and/or steak works well, especially if marinated in teriyaki sauce and served with lemon zest seasoning and twice-baked potato. Throw in a glass of finely aged Merlot and soon you'll forget you were ever injured. But I digress.

Compression means wrapping the affected area. This can be done with athletic tape or various braces or splints. Consult your physician to see what would be the best approach.

Elevation means raising the affected area above your heart. The idea is to help gravity drain some of the fluid from the area, thereby reducing the swelling. If the strained area is the gas tank of that pesky neighbor whose dog keeps fertilizing your lawn, and the heart is the container you're going to use to siphon gas out of his tank, the procedure only works if the container is lower than the chassis (or so I'm told). So our weekend warrior would lie on the ground and prop his ailing ankle on the couch and desperately try to pry sympathy out of his wife. (Did I mention this is all hypothetical?)

So the next time you're up at 6 a.m. watching the clash between South Korea and Togo and you notice the trainer giving an ever-so-subtle wink at the camera, you'll know exactly what he means. Their secret's safe with us. Go team!

Medicare Drug Cards

I have a deck of cards that I got from the Paris Las Vegas hotel in—not France. I like it quite a lot. It's shiny, springy and easy to hold. I've played solitaire with it, built flimsy houses, and at times lost money to friends with it. But that will be nothing compared to the deck being dealt by Medicare.

Yes, the Medicare Modernization Act (MMA) (is it just me or does that acronym sound awfully maternal?) moves on to part D. (The 'D' stands for 'Dang, these medications are expensive! Somebody help me!') This means that very soon, if not already, Medicare subscribers will start receiving mail, phone calls, emails, telegrams, singing telegrams, flying banners, and creatively carved hedges inviting them to sign up with the advertiser for the Medicare Drug Card. What a far cry this is from the days when finding prescription coverage for seniors was like trying to find an employee at the Home Depot. The difference? You guessed it—money! That eternally powerful motivator that makes the world go 'round. Now that there's money to be made, insurance companies can't wait to cover your drugs.

Medicare could have taken on this responsibility, but instead chose to go the free-market route. Because otherwise it'd be socialized medicine and we might as well wear berets and striped t-shirts and sit in cafes saying, 'Je voudrais un café', which means, 'We 'ave universal 'ealthcare.' Besides, like insurance and drug companies have clearly shown us, in the free-market model of healthcare, the patient wins!

The plan is very simple. Allow me to paraphrase:

The party henceforth known as the 'principle party' shall set forth, contingent upon their agreement, medications—henceforth referred to as 'bait'—to supply the client henceforth referred to as 'client' with goods and services agreed upon hereto by the above, exempting inclusions. The client on his/her part agrees forthwith to gather funds for such 'bait', effective upon completion of the pre-determined optional but recommended monetary levy including but not limited to the limitations. The client also agrees to the terms and conditions of the periodic requisitions as set forth by the principle party. The client and principle party may not agree to disagree unless agreed upon by previous disagreements or disagreed upon by previous agreements.

In other words, seniors get to choose what card they buy. It'll cost about $30 a month. The insurance company decides which medications to provide. So how will you know which is the right card for you among the 2,654,448.35 being offered? Easy. Just go to *www.medicare.gov* and use the friendly guide. Not comfortable with a computer? No problem, just call 1-800-Medicare and qualified automated assistants will assist you. Not comfortable with the phone? No problem. Just go to the local Social Security Office. Not comfortable meeting in person? Then perhaps you should consider medications for Social Anxiety Disorder. Of course, the irony is that you need to sign up for a plan in order to get the medication.

In most cases, the subscriber is responsible for the first $250 of the medication. From then on, the plan covers up to $2250 a year (there might be a co-pay). From $2250 to about $3600, the patient pays for the entire amount. After $3600, the plan covers 95 percent of the cost of the medications.

But what if you're one of the five seniors nationwide who is only taking one or two medications and they're all generic? Don't worry. Medicare has thought of you, too. For every year you don't enroll, you get penalized in the form of higher monthly payments for a program when you *do* sign up. So, it might be best to sign up while the getting's good.

Who's paying for this? Why, we all are! Medicare will give insurance companies hundreds of billions of dollars a year for the coverage.

You can change plans if you so choose but only in the open enrollment period which runs November through December of each year—right around the holidays when it's nice and quiet and there are no large family gatherings or frantic shopping binges.

So gather your list of medications and go fish!

A Message from the Gut

Greetings, reader! This is your stomach speaking. Thanks for the ice cream last night. I wasn't sure how it would go with the pickled herring and peanut butter, but we managed to keep everyone in for the night.

From all the cold desserts and drinks that have been coming in as of late, I'm surmising that it must be summertime. Since we live in a coastal city, winding up on a boat is inevitable. Summertime also brings with it long car rides and plane flights. You might have noticed that some of these don't quite settle well with me.

Allow me to explain: This is not my fault. I am absolutely innocent. The provocateur is the brain. That's right, the high-and-mighty-I'm-the-seat-of-consciousness organ that sits in its ivory, bone-enforced castle on top of the neck while us visceral organs are left here with nothing but some flimsy muscle tissue to protect us. Yet, deprive the brain of sugar for just a few minutes and it starts to fall apart. And guess who's responsible for putting sugar into the blood stream so the brain can use it? Yours truly. But I'm not bitter. Like my therapist always tells me (breathe in), 'This is a team effort. It takes all the organs working together to make the body work' (aaaaannd breathe out).

Anyway, I'm bound by orders from the brain. It tells me to work harder or slow down or send things back. When you embark on these voyages, we sense the rocking, turning, and dipping in here. And we don't mind. Sometimes it's even fun. It helps to break the monotony of intestinal gurgling. Believe me, I tell it to keep it down during those intensely silent moments, but it has a mind of its own. Besides, it's so long, that by the time the message gets to the other end, it's too late and we've already made a bit of a scene.

But I digress.

So we feel the movements, but so does your inner-ear balance centers. The problem arises when your eyes don't agree with the inner ear. The brain gets mixed signals. It's not unlike the kids sometimes in the back seat: 'We're rocking.' 'No we're not.' 'Yes, we are.' 'No we're not!' 'Yes we are!!' 'NO WE'RE NOT!!'. Then the brain flips out. Much like when you tell the kids, 'Don't make me stop this car!' the brain, in its own language, expresses its frustration. Part of that language involves sending a signal to me to stop all digestion. So we sit and wait for the eyes and the inner ear to sort it out. As we all know, food is only good for a short time, especially in the stomach. So when the time runs out, we can't keep the food anymore and so we send it back. To look on the positive side, I've heard that it attracts fish. (Don't ask me how I know that. It's a long story.)

The best way to solve the bickering of the eyes and the inner ear is to help the eyes to confirm that the body's moving. Looking at the road when in a car, looking at a fixed point on the horizon when on a boat, looking out the window when in a plane can all help.

There's also medication available to calm things down. There are patches and pills. They work in some people. But the drawback is that they can give some people a dry mouth or make them sleepy.

That's all I have to say. Thank you for listening. I've been meaning to get that off my—chest (so to speak) for quite a while. Don't tell the eyes and the inner ear that I ratted them out. You thought I was sensitive—don't get those two started!!

Migraines, Your Grains,
It Doesn't Matter—My Head
Still Hurts

Having a migraine is like having a baby or going to medical school: it's impossible to know what it's like until one has gone through it. But unlike medical school, once a migraine starts, it's not too late to do something about it. For some people, having children and going to medical school can cause migraines. Maybe having migraines has driven some people to medical school where they meet their soul mate and wind up having children who exacerbate their migraines? If medical schools started having children, then I think we would all get migraines.

But I digress.

A migraine is a very special kind of headache. 'Special' in the same way that a hurricane is a 'special' rainstorm. A hurricane has enormous destructive power—whether it's in the bay off of New Orleans, or in a large plastic cup on Bourbon Street. Migraines have a similarly destructive power.

A number of characteristics makes migraines unique. One aspect is the intensity of the pain. If a regular headache hurts like getting punched in the arm by a friend who has spotted a 'slugbug', a migraine hurts like being hit on the arm by a giant demolition ball.

The other aspect that distinguishes a migraine from a regular headache is its entourage. If a regular headache is like Joe Public going grocery shopping all by himself, a migraine is like the President going on a diplomatic mission to a foreign land, complete with Vice President Nausea, Assistant Vice President Vomiting (those two sure know how to kill a diplomatic party!), and Secretary of the Department of Sensitivity to Light and Sound. If the trip is really intense, the Head of Homeland Stroke-Like Symptoms might go, too.

Due to the entourage of bonus symptoms described above, migraine sufferers tend to seek out dark, quiet places to rest. A neurologist once described migraines as a 'hibernating phenomena' meaning that it triggers 'hibernating' behavior in humans. Perhaps that is why bears hibernate—they're having a three-month long migraine. No wonder they can be cranky. Perhaps, instead of playing dead, we should carry migraine medicine when roaming the woods . . . just in case.

Any stress on the body can trigger a migraine. Not sleeping enough or over sleeping, sun exposure, certain foods, and stressful life situations can all trigger migraines. In women, periods can cause migraines.

These days, migraine sufferers don't have to hibernate if they don't want to. There are medications that can help treat migraines. Ibuprofen (Advil, Motrin) in high enough doses can be effective. Combination acetaminophen, aspirin and caffeine tablets (Excedrin) can be effective as well. There are also a multitude of prescription medications for treating acute migraines and preventing recurrences, such as sumatriptan (Imitrex), Tylenol with codeine, and naratriptan (Amerge). But the trick is to take the medication early in the course of the migraine—the sooner it is taken, the better it works. Once a migraine is established and going full force, it can be hard to break.

So if there are people out there who get headaches that interfere with their lives, bring with them an entourage of bonus symptoms, and make them want to find a dark, quiet place to rest, the headaches might be migraines. Consider a visit with your healthcare provider to clarify the diagnosis and start treatment, if appropriate. Also, since certain events can trigger a migraine, keeping a headache diary can help determine a pattern. Things to note are when the migraine occured, the components and timing of the most recent meal, how much sleep was attained the previous night, and anything else that seems noteworthy. One need not list medical school or having children since those are non-modifiable risk factors.

The Morning After
the Night Before

Like the Yeti of the Himalayas, the Sasquatch of the Americas and the Lochness Monster of Scotland, so has the Morning After Pill long lived in legend. There have been numerous sightings. There have been people who know people who know people whose cousin's ex-girlfriend's neighbor once saw one. There have even been blurry photographs and grainy video footage—most of which eventually turned out to be hoaxes. Join me today in this undercover report to discover the truths, the myths, and unravel the mystery of: 'The Morning After Pill—Damnation or Salvation'.

When I was a young(er) man, I had heard vaguely about a pill that could be used to prevent what I considered at that time to be pure disaster—worse than the Titanic, the Hindenburg, and Kelly Clarkson's movie combined. I can't tell you from whom I heard it. It's just one of those things that I came to know. I came to like the other gender much in the same way. I don't know exactly when it happened. I just know that one day I stopped seeing girls as walking masses of highly contagious and infectious cooties and saw them as beings that evoked my curiosity and magically took away all of my verbal skills and made me want to vomit. Those were troubled, lonely years.

Fortunately, I got over my vomiting Neanderthal routine by the time I was 21, and found myself involved in a relationship. One day I actually had to inquire about the Morning After Pill. If it existed, it would be more precious to me than all the tea in Fort Knox. Since I definitely had not Planned on becoming a Parent anytime soon, I turned to the be-all-end-all of family planning: Planned Parenthood. The answer I got from the receptionist was very vague. She basically said that my partner would have to come in for an exam before they could answer any of my questions. She never did go for the exam and, fortunately, we did not become Parents as we had not Planned. But that sure was a long week!

So naturally, when I went to medical school and started to study gynecology and reproductive stuff, I was very curious about this Morning After Pill. I came to realize that indeed it does exist. Yes, you've read correctly. I'm stating loud and clear for the whole world to hear. I shall shout it from the mountain top! Tell your friends! Tell your neighbors! Tell your neighbor's children to tell your children! There IS a Morning After Pill and it's fabulous! It can be up to 95+ percent effective, if taken in time. You can take it up to five days after 'the night before', but it's much more effective the earlier it is taken. Some women are so pro-active and involved in Planning their Parenthood that they have some on hand—just in case—so that there are no delays.

The Morning After Pill is beautifully simple in design. It's basically a whopping dose of birth-control pills taken 12 hours apart. Like most things of simple beauty, we don't know exactly how it works. It most likely changes the uterus such that the fertilized egg does not implant. But we *do* know that if a pregnancy has already occurred, it will not abort it.

Its safety is impeccable. Nausea and irregular bleeding are the main side effects and they're temporary. There are no long-term health problems with the Morning After Pill. In fact, it is so safe and effective that there is some talk about letting pharmacists dispense it without a prescription. But as it stands now, you need a doctor's prescription.

But, like all birth control pills, the Morning After Pill does not protect against sexually transmitted diseases. It only prevents pregnancy.

So all you people out there not Planning on becoming Parents, here's another option to keep the Plan alive. Here again is my favorite line from pharmaceutical ads: Talk to your doctor to see if the Morning After Pill is right for you. It's never too early to have *that* discussion.

For those parents of teens out there and for the few teens that might be reading this, consider opening some dialogue. Sure, it's about as comfortable as the nightmare where you show up for school in your underwear, but it might beat the alternative.

New Year, Less Money, Same Body Part I

My apologies to my faithful readers, mom and dad, for my long hiatus over the holidays. Now I'm back with more jibber-jabber, so listen up!

It's no secret that we are the richest nation in the history of the world. It's also no secret that we're the heaviest nation in the history of the world. Many brave individuals have pledged to do something about it with the New Year. Usually this means a gym membership that gets used until Valentine's Day, or an expensive, bulky piece of exercise equipment that eventually becomes a pricy clothes rack.

Exercise commitments usually bring along with them their good buddy, the diet. Everybody has their favorite: Atkins, South Beach, Mediterranean, low-fat, the Zone, and on and on.

Unfortunately, despite their good intentions, most people wind up regaining any lost weight and sometimes more. So where do these well-intentioned men and women go wrong? Everybody has their own theory and here's my own unfounded and highly biased version.

FACT: Being overweight is a result of longstanding (usually lifelong) habits.

Imagine your body as a bank account: If every day you take in $1 more in calories than you burn, in 10 years you'll have over $3650 of extra calories in your body. Your body keeps these extra calories in a 'safe' around the waist and thighs.

FACT: Habits are very hard to change in the long run. I believe most people's attempts at diet and exercise are too drastic of a change from their norm and therefore impossible to maintain. Over time, they slip back into the same habits that made them overweight in the first place.

It's like the frog in the pot analogy: If you put a frog in a pot of hot water, it will jump out. But if you put a frog in a pot of room temperature water and slowly heat it up, the frog will stay in and the next thing you know, dinner is served. (I hear it's great with horseradish.)

Turning on the diet and exercise heat slowly makes for a more sustainable change. Try starting with a food diary. List everything you eat for a week. Just looking at the list can sometimes give some very helpful hints. Then, commit to making a small change each week or month, however you're comfortable. Keep the changes small. For example, instead of drinking two regular sodas a day, drink one regular and one diet.

Liquids are a very common source of extra calories. Juices, sodas, sports drinks and anything besides water and non-fat milk have lots of extra calories.

A reasonable starting weight loss goal is 10 percent over the first year. Yes, it's slow, but it's sustainable. You probably won't be modeling in any men's or women's swimsuit catalogs by the summer, but it'll be a start.

Furthermore, people who have lost weight and kept it off have a few traits in common. They all eat breakfast every day. They follow a low-fat high *complex* carbohydrate diet (whole wheat bread, whole oats, etc.).

So be diligent in your efforts, brave men and women. The marathon of weight loss starts with the very first step.

New Year, Less Money, Same Body Part II

Now is the time to get 'money back' on the 'money back guarantee' of the muscle-building-fat-burning-glute-shaping-peck-defining machine that folds and fits neatly under the bed. Unless, of course, you actually *use* the machine for its intended purpose.

People often ask, 'How much exercise should I do?' The National Institute of Health's response is, '60 minutes of moderate activity a day.' The average person, upon hearing this, throws their hands in the air, slumps on the couch, and reaches for the remote control. Shane Murphy, PhD, author of the book 'The Achievement Zone', brings up a very good point. If you have to ask the question, you're not doing the right kind of exercise. He argues that any activity in which one partakes should be fun. And if it is, then you would naturally do plenty of it. So for all those out there counting minutes until they're done with their workouts and dreading the next, why not try something else?

Essentially, 'activity' means anything that involves movement. It doesn't necessarily have to be walking or weights. Housework is activity. Dancing, any style and no matter how bad, is activity. Home improvement projects, swimming, looking for your car keys, and pushing a shopping cart around the grocery store are all activities. So, experiment. Find something you like.

An easy way to keep track of activity level is to get a pedometer. It's a small device, about the size of a pager, that clips on to your belt. It counts how many steps you take. You can find them in most fitness stores and they cost about $20. Wear it to see how many steps you take in an average day. Then, try to increase that number by 1,000 steps a day each month, until you're taking 10,000 steps a day. It seems like a daunting number, but it's not. Little things here and there can really add to the total: Parking a few spaces further away, getting up to turn off the TV, taking stairs instead of elevators, all add hundreds, if not thousands, of steps every day.

As mentioned earlier, the key is to make small changes. It probably won't get you back into your high school prom tuxedo or gown (if you weighed less in high school), but at the very least it will keep your weight from increasing, which is *very* important from a medical standpoint. It could also help you lose the 10 percent over the first year that we discussed before.

Some people ask what their ideal weight should be. For this, we have our friendly BMI: the Body Mass Index. It's a reliable indicator of overall body fat and will tell you if you're at risk of future health problems from your weight.

It's a fairly simple calculation. So get out your calculators and follow these simple instructions:

> *Enter your weight in pounds.*
> *Hit the divide key* (the dash with dots above and below it)
> *Enter your height in inches.*
> *Hit the divide key* (see above)
> *Enter your height in inches, again.*
> *Hit the multiply key* (X)
> *Enter 703*
> *Hit the equal key* (=)

If the number you got is between 20 and 24.9, you're in good shape. Don't change a thing. If your number is between 25 and 29.9, you are in the 'overweight range'. The important thing here is to keep your weight from *increasing*. Sure, weight loss is great, but it's just as important not to gain. If your number is above 30.0, you are in the 'obese' range. This means that you are at risk of health problems, such as diabetes, high blood pressure, arthritis, and heart disease from your weight. You should consult your doctor.

There is one caveat with the BMI. People who are muscular will have a high BMI and not necessarily be 'overweight' or 'obese'. To help sort out these gubernatorial-types, we measure the waist size. No, not the number on the tag inside your pants, but the 'medical' waist size, which is the smallest measurement around the belly measured below the ribs and above the belly button. A number above 40 for men and 35 for women means that it's not just the bulging biceps that are elevating the BMI.

The Pain of Pain Relief

I imagine Lance Armstrong wakes up after winning the Tour de France with some aches and pains. I also imagine that he treks down to his local drugstore to look for some relief. Of course, in reality, he probably has a personal physician at his beck and call and the drugstore delivers anything he wants directly to his door by moped, ironically. But for the sake of argument, let's pretend he actually has to go there himself.

Once there, he gets accosted by a battalion of bottles and packages all desperately vying for his attention. The 'fat cats' of over-the-counter pain medications, like Advil, Aleve, and Tylenol, occupy the prime, eye-level real estate. The lesser known brands are forced to look up from their peon levels and dream of climbing these shelves of success. Perhaps he sees his picture on a bottle of the 'FRS' supplement he promotes and wonders if his nose is really that crooked?

Trying to choose the right pain reliever can be a pain in and of itself. There are tablets, capsules, gelcaps, and melt-in-your-mouth-not-in-your-gym-bag redi-tabs. There are boxes, child-proof bottles that require a three-year-old to open, and regular bottles that still require a three-year-old to open. So how is a sore Tour de France winner to choose the right medication?

The truth is that there hasn't been a breakthrough in over-the-counter medication for thirteen years. Basically, there are anti-inflammatories (ibuprofen, naproxen, and aspirin) and acetaminophen (Tylenol).

The benefit of anti-inflammatories is that, as the name suggests, they can help reduce inflammation which is the most common cause of pain associated with exercise. By reducing inflammation, they not only control pain, but can also promote healing.

We don't really know what acetaminophen does. We know it does not reduce inflammation, so it won't help anything heal more quickly. We do know that it relieves pain, although we're not sure exactly how. We also know that it is one of the safest medications out there. It hardly interacts with anything and only if someone has liver failure should they be careful when taking it. But it's not a very strong pain reliever. That's why it likes to buddy-up with big gun opiates like hydrocodone and oxycodone to make Vicodin and Percocet.

In fact, acetaminophen and anti-inflammatories can be taken together since they work in completely different ways. It's an easy way to boost the pain-relieving effect of either one.

Then why do we have so many different brands when there are really only four active ingredients? Why *money*, of course! In the free market, if there isn't a new product in the field, repackage the old ones and advertise! It's a great deal. The active ingredients (the anti-inflammatories and acetaminophen) are dirt cheap. One can buy a 500,000 count bottle at Costco for 49 cents. So repackage it under a brand name and sell fifty pills for six dollars. Try it at home!

So my advice to Lance is, if you have a favorite pain reliever, look at the active ingredient on the box, and next time, just purchase the active ingredient. It'll be the exact same medication but a lot less expensive. (Unless you have a strong attachment to the packaging and colorful letters on the pills.) If you do not have a favorite pain reliever, and are otherwise healthy, consider using an anti-inflammatory medication. Not only will it help with the pain, but it might get you back on the bike sooner. You can use acetaminophen as an add-on, if needed.

Good luck, and hope you get well soon.

Maybe you should have stuck with Sheryl after all!

The Party Bug

The FIFA World Cup is over for now. Soccer fever was everywhere! From the small towns in middle America to the big cities on the coasts, fans of all ages were up at 4:30 in the morning, tuning in via television, Internet, cell phone, iPad and dramatic re-enactment to watch New Zealand take on Slovakia (or insert your favorite teams).

The World Cup took place in South Africa this time around. Every night in South Africa there was much revelry by winners celebrating a victory, losers coping with grief and impartial fans looking for any excuse to revel. But humans aren't the only ones revelling in the evenings. Like every other part of the world (with the possible exception of Antarctica), mosquitoes are revelling in the evenings as well.

In South Africa's case, some of those mosquitoes are carrying revellers of their own, the malaria bug. The malaria bug is a protozoan, which means that it is a more complex, aka 'evolved', organism than bacteria and viruses. (And I hear it takes every opportunity to rub our bacterial and viral noses in it, too!)

When it's not taunting lower life forms, the malaria bug looks for humans to infect. When a mosquito stings a human, it inserts its long, needle-like nose into the skin looking to hit a vein. The malaria bugs stand by with their bags packed and little ones in tow, threatening to leave them behind if they don't stop poking their sister. When the mosquito's nose hits a vein, they run like gangbusters down the mosquito's nose and into the human circulation, leaving behind a trail of loose papers and a child's shoe.

Once inside the human body, the malaria bug relaxes, stretches, and unpacks. The human body is a very desirable place for malaria bugs. The accommodations are first class and food is readily available in the form of human red blood cells. Naturally, when the immediate needs of food and housing are met, the malaria bug turns to procreation.

After procreation, the malaria bug looks to infect other humans. Since its one and only mode of transportation is the mosquito, this presents a challenge: How can they predict when their human host is going to get stung by a mosquito again? Apparently, the malaria bug has had a long time to think about this problem because it has come up with a reasonable solution.

Since mosquitoes tend to come out at night, the malaria bug follows suit. Every evening, the malaria bug family packs its bags once again, and once again threatens to leave the kids behind if it hears one more complaint about having to move again! And how should it know where the crayons are? It doesn't use them.

Then the malaria bug family moves out into the circulation to find a mosquito nose. When it does, they run like gangbusters again to get back into the mosquito and the cycle starts all over again. The malaria bugs that don't find a mosquito nose go back into hiding until the next night.

When the malaria bug moves out into the blood stream, the immune system sounds the 'intruder alert' alarm and tries to kill off the malaria bugs. People who are infected with malaria experience this as fever, chills, and body aches. When the malaria bugs go back into hiding, the immune system sounds the 'all clear' bell and the fever, chills, and body aches go away. This gives malaria its classic 'cyclical fever': patients feel very ill in the evenings, yet feel remarkably better in the morning, only to have the symptoms come back in the evening again.

There are medications available to treat malaria. The same medications can also *prevent* malaria if taken prior to, during, and after travel. So hopefully all the revellers in South Africa took their malaria-preventing medications. And hopefully they've used insect repellent and avoided being outdoors at sunset to reduce mosquito bites as a further precaution, so they can stay malaria-free and look forward to the next World Cup!

Patellofemoral Pain Syndrome

What would we do without our knees? Religious institutions would have to get creative in how people show devotion. Rock stars would have to glide across the stage in roller shoes instead of doing the more dramatic knee slide. And the traditional marriage proposal would be a man doing the splits before his beloved, which could wind up delaying many a nuptial.

But thankfully, we do have knees. And like most other body parts, one does not realize how much one needs them until they get injured. I don't know what the exact prevalence of knee injuries is but I would bet that any given person has fewer degrees of separation from someone with knee problems than a Kevin Bacon movie.

Among knee injuries, ACL (Anterior Cruciate Ligament) tears are the rock stars. They tend to hang around celebrity athletes. They receive state-of-the-art surgical treatments involving the moving of tendons from other parts of the body or using the ACLs of people who won't be using them anymore. And afterwards, they require a lot of physical therapy and rehabilitation.

On the other end of the spectrum is patellofemoral pain syndrome. It can occur in working class people. It has no surgical treatment and can drag out for months, if not years.

'Patello' refers to the patella, aka knee cap. 'Femoral' refers to the femur, aka thigh bone. 'Pain' is a noxious stimulus. (This is not to be confused with an *obnoxious* stimulus, such as the cast of Glee doing their rendition of 'Somebody to Love' by Queen. I'm not sure which is worse: months and months of nagging knee pain or four minutes and forty-three seconds of heartless over-singing of a classic. But I digress.)

To understand the cause of patellofemoral pain syndrome, we must first review the normal workings of the knee cap. The knee cap moves up and down as the knee bends and straightens. The cartilage under the knee cap is V-shaped and sits on a groove on the thigh bone. If we think of the knee cap as an unruly toddler, the groove would be the water slide down which one would carefully guide said toddler to show her how much 'fun' it is.

The thigh muscles help the knee cap move smoothly down the center of the groove. One set of muscles pulls the knee cap from the right, and another set pulls it from the left. It's like mommy and daddy each grabbing one of the toddler's arms and guiding her down the water slide. If mommy and daddy are equally strong, the toddler glides right down the middle of the slide, happy as can be and squealing in delight until water gets in her eyes, at which point she screams bloody murder and will have to be subdued with chocolate milk.

But if daddy is more eager than mommy, the toddler gets dragged to one side, ruining the smooth ride and prompting more chocolate milk bribery. The same thing can happen to the knee caps of runners and people who have to do a lot of kneeling and squatting, such as mechanics, housekeepers, and plumbers. Over time, the thigh muscles on one side get stronger than the other, ruining the knee cap's smooth glide and causing inflammation and pain.

People experience this as pain under the knee cap that is worse with kneeling, running, or standing after prolonged sitting. Anti-inflammatories, physical therapy, and activity modification can get the muscles equally strong once again, but it can take months of diligence and perseverence with the program to yield results.

In other words, the story of how one became afflicted with patellofemoral pain syndrome won't make a good ice breaker at a singles event, but the story of the recovery could be an epic tale to rival any water park thrill ride, provided there are no star athletes recovering from ACL surgery in the room.

Phlegmsnot

If our respiratory secretions were a celebrity couple, one of whom was a furiously devout Scientologist and the other a teen star who, through the years, has blossomed into a fine young lady and mother and we can't see what she possibly sees in him except for his stunning good looks, storybook career, and wealth beyond my wildest dreams—what was I talking about? Oh yes, if our respiratory secretions were a celebrity couple like the one above, the tabloids would refer to them as 'Phlegmsnot'

'Phlegm' is the common term for mucus coughed up from the lungs. 'Snot' is the common term for mucus coming down from the nose. With cold and flu season approaching the All-Star break, many people have had about as much phlegmsnot as they can handle and are looking desperately for some fresh Lindsay Lohan gossip to break the monotony.

But how does one make phlegmsnot go away?

I'm afraid the answer is rather unexciting and certainly not glamorous: Time.

Most phlegmsnot will go away with time no matter what we do. But that doesn't mean that we simply roll over and wait. Some of us fight with valor to the slimy, salty end. We blow our noses until we pop blood vessels in our eyes which give us that spooky horror-movie look. We cough and cough until our faces turn red to complement our eyes.

Some of us take to the local drugstore where, thanks to the pharmaceutical industry, we can try a different phlegmsnot-fighting medication every day of the month and never repeat. It's variety that would make Rachael Ray sit up and take notice!

Then there's the spit vs. swallow controversy. Spitting is not only socially frowned upon, but it can spread the infection. On the other hand, there is the intense satisfaction of knowing that we've gotten at least some part of the illness physically out of our bodies.

Some fear that by swallowing phlegmsnot, they're making the infection last longer. Nothing could be further from the truth. Once swallowed, the stomach acid effectively kills any and all bugs, rendering the phlegmsnot sterile. The intestines then digest it without blinking an eye. The entire lining of the stomach is already covered with mucus so the stomach barely notices the difference.

Then there's the matter of the phlegmsnot that sits in the airways hanging on for dear life. No force of nature seems to be able to dislodge it. That's when our amazing bodies come to the rescue. Amazingly, once the disease has run its course, whatever phlegmsnot is not expelled or swallowed gets sucked back in through the walls of the nose or the air passageways in the lungs. It's true! The very same entities that produce the phlegmsnot actually take it back! (No questions asked! No receipt necessary! No restrictions! Thank you for shopping at the respiratory system! Please come back soon!)

So as we all battle phlegmsnot next cold and flu season, let's make sure to do all the things that will help us get well: rest, drink plenty of fluids, and try a decongestant to help prevent a sinus infection. Let's also do all the things that keep our phlegmsnot from spreading to other victims, such as covering our coughs and finding appropriate places to dispose of our expelled phlegmsnot. One thing that we need not worry about is swallowing it or being able to cough it all up or blow it all out or . . . . Our bodies have us covered for that. And perhaps the next time we're in the grocery store, we'll feel brave enough to scan the cover of Time magazine—provided there 's no fresh 'Brangelina' dirt to be found.

The Piggy Flu aka H1N1

A close look at any 'street' interview on the news will show a microscopic virus jumping up and down in the background vying for screen time. Why, it seems like just a few weeks ago, we had apocalyptic visions of deserted urban landscapes where a lone man and his dog fight off infected zombies who come out at night to feed on human flesh. The movie version would star Will Smith as the lone man and, since he loves listening to Frank Sinatra, it would be called, 'I Am Blue Eyes (When Wearing Colored Contacts)'.

But I digress.

So the swine flu gave the world a pretty big scare. Actually, the pig farmers of America don't want us to call it swine flu since, technically, it is made up of swine, avian and human flu parts. So now it is known as the H1N1 flu which sounds rather dry and technical. I think 'Piggy Flu' has a better ring to it. Or 'Chimera flu' for something a little more exotic. Why not 'Flu Out the Window' just to work in a play on words?

So the swine flu, aka 'H1N1 flu', had all the elements of our worst public health nightmare: a virus that normally lives in other animals making the jump to humans and then spreading from human to human. Since it would be a brand new virus for humans, our immune systems would be slow to react and that would put us at higher risk of becoming gravely ill or dying.

As it turns out, the swine flu hasn't quite been the doomsday bug we first thought. But it has served as a good exercise for our global pandemic response.

The first step in any pandemic is identifying the people who have the disease. In the case of the swine flu, we knew that its symptoms were similar to human flu, so how were we to tell them apart? To help make the distinction, a test was developed to detect the swine flu. But our ability to run the test was quickly overwhelmed by the number of samples submitted and so local Public Health Departments had to prioritize which samples to run first. This left a lot of people not knowing if they had the swine flu or the seasonal flu.

The second part is keeping the people who have the disease from giving it to other people. Since the swine flu seems to spread in the same way as human flu, the recommendation is for people to stay home if they have flu-like symptoms—just to be safe. The general population should cover their coughs and wash their hands regularly. This way, even if there is someone with the swine flu who has not been tested or is awaiting results, at least he/she would not infect other people.

The third part is trying to stay one step ahead of the pandemic by continuously updating recommendations for screening and treatment. The World Health Organization (WHO), the Center for Disease Control (CDC) and local Public Health Agencies all had to work together and share information to keep track of the illness. For the most part, it seems like this was done fairly effectively since it seemed like every hour a new country would report confirmed swine flu cases.

The more effectively we can accomplish these three steps, the better we will deal with any pandemic. So far, the swine flu hasn't been any more deadly than the seasonal flu so the consequences of any missteps haven't been so dire. But let's hope the world governments seize this opportunity to work out any kinks such that, if and when the next pandemic occurs, our response will be swifter and more effective.

Until then, these websites can provide us with updated information on the current swine flu aka H1N1 pandemic.

For global status, *www.who.int*

For national updates, *www.cdc.gov/h1n1*

For local updates, *www.sbcphd.org*

Happy surfing.

The Piggy Flu Shot

As you, the conscientious, intelligent, and disarmingly sweet-smelling reader are reading these words, millions of doses of the Novel H1N1 Flu, aka swine flu, vaccine are making their way across the country. If one listens closely, one can hear the lack of sound coming from the Styrofoam-insulated boxes. It was hoped that the vaccine would make it into people's deltoids before October 4, the official start of flu season, but we've clearly missed that mark.

School-aged children are already back in close quarters, sharing snot and saliva. And since they are the ones at highest risk of getting the swine flu, there is an urgency to get a large number of people vaccinated in a rather short period of time.

That task is further complicated by some people's mistrust of the safety of a vaccine that apparently has been rushed to market. Many people are wondering if we know enough about the long-term consequences of this new vaccine to give it to so many people.

But the reality is that this vaccine isn't actually that new. It is identical in every way to the seasonal flu vaccine that has been around for decades. It is made in the same facilities with the same machines, the same recipe, and the same people wearing the same lab coats as the seasonal flu. (Except perhaps their badges read 'SHNU'—Special H1N1 Unit.)

Besides that, the only difference between the Novel H1N1 vaccine and the seasonal flu vaccine is the virus pieces. It's like taking grandma's spinach lasagna recipe and in Step 23 adding green bell peppers instead of red bell peppers. In the end, the difference will be slight, and the lasagna will be just as safe to consume (assuming one consumed it in the first place and did not feed it to the dog under the table, ever vigilant not to get caught for fear of inciting another story about the Great Depression. But I digress.)

The Novel H1N1 flu vaccine has been tested in over 4500 subjects so far. None of them has had any serious side effects besides soreness at the injection site and low-grade fevers for a day or so. So we can say that the chances of a serious side effect from this new vaccine will be at least less than one in 4500. To put that in perspective, the odds of getting injured from mowing the lawn are one in 3600. (I'm still working on getting hazard pay from my wife.) The odds of fatally slipping in a bath or shower are one in 2200.

The other thing to keep in mind as the H1N1 flu gets administered is that bad things happen all the time. If a bad event happens after getting the H1N1 flu vaccine, the first question would be, is it coincidence, or related to the vaccine? To answer that question, one must compare the rate of the possible event in the vaccine population to that of the general population.

For example, let's assume that the rate of eye twitching in the general population is one percent. If public health departments get calls from people complaining of eye twitches after receiving the Novel H1N1 vaccine, they will compare that to the rate of eye twitching in the general population. If the rate of eye twitching in the vaccine group is also one percent, then it is unlikely that the eye twitching is from the vaccine. If the rate of eye twitching in the vaccine group is five percent, then the vaccine might be causing twitching. If the rate of eye twitching is less than one percent in the vaccine group then the vaccine might somehow cure twitchy eyes.

So if one is willing to risk taking a shower before going to get the H1N1 flu vaccine, the riskiest part of the day will already be over. However, regardless of whether one chooses to get vaccinated or not, it is still very important to wash hands, cover coughs and sneezes with elbows, and stay home from work or school if one gets flu-like symptoms. That will be our best bet at keeping the seasonal flu and the H1N1 flu at bay—short of hiding in a bomb shelter until Spring.

Preventing Relapses

As I see it, there are two types of resolutions: personal and UN. Personal resolutions tend to be a call to action to change a behavior and there is usually a big surge of them around the New Year. A UN resolution, on the other hand, does not follow a seasonal pattern. It's when all the countries in the world get together and set aside their similarities in order to come to a disagreement on a global issue. If they fail to disagree, then one of the G8 nations will help out with a veto. The 'G8' are the nations that have found regular UN classes not challenging enough and thus are placed in an advanced placement, or 'gate' class. It's spelled 'G8' because texting is huge in the UN.

But I digress.

Any individual trying to change a behavior goes through four stages: 'Pre-contemplative', 'Contemplative', 'Action', and 'Maintenance'. As an example, let's consider the case of a hypothetical physician writer who has decided to stop wearing hole-y socks (meaning socks with holes in them, not socks that have been granted sainthood).

Our hypothetical physician, let's call him Dr. J, would have started in the 'Pre-contemplative' phase. In this phase, he wouldn't see any sock problem. He wouldn't even think about changing anything. When people would comment on his socks, he would tell them that he enjoys holes in his socks and that he actually needs the air circulation to keep his feet cool and fungus free.

Then he would start thinking that perhaps it would be nice not to have to pull forward the end of his sock and stuff it in between his toes only to have the great toe stick its head out like some podiatric tortoise. But even though he thought about it, he wouldn't be quite ready to do anything. That would be his 'Contemplative' phase.

But on December 31, he would enter his 'Action phase'. He'd have done his thinking and would be ready to act! He would toss out all his hole-y socks and start fresh with intact footwear. That would put him in the fourth stage of change, 'Maintenance'. The key in the Maintenance phase is to prevent a relapse.

Lord knows many are the times that Dr. J tried to stop wearing hole-y socks. But when the tip of the sock started to fade, he would think to himself, 'Well that's no reason to toss out a perfectly good pair of socks. I've still got time.' When he would start to see the outline of his great toe through the disintegrating fabric, he would think, 'It's not technically a *hole*. No reason to throw away a fairly good pair of socks.' Then the nail would start to stick out. 'Well, I'll only wear those socks when I know I won't be taking my shoes off in public' would be his typical excuse.

And the next thing he knows, half the socks in his drawer have holes in them again.

But looking on the bright side, each one of those failed attempts was a learning experience. This time he's well armed and his chances of success are better than ever! He shall look back and see what worked and what didn't work and try to avoid some of his previous pitfalls.

So this year, as we all try to get maximum vice time in before the New Year, let's take reassurance in the fact that just by having made a resolution, we have completed three out of the four stages of change. Most of the work is already done. At this point, some reflection on what was difficult about continuing previous resolutions and experimenting with things to do when a relapse-causing situation arises can greatly improve our chances of success.

So Happy New Year to all resoluters and otherwise. And no matter what happens with our resolutions, at least we have the UN to make us look good.

Probiotic

Picture an amateur biotic who has just landed a five-year contract worth $144 million. Imagine someone standing outside Congress holding a sign that says, 'Biotics have rights, too' while a new bill regarding antibiotics is on the floor.

Neither of the above cases is a probiotic. However, probiotics can be found in bottles in certain stores.

If I were doing an infomercial for a probiotic company, I would run it thus: Picture me in a long white coat, standing in an official-looking office with lots of books on the walls. Maybe I'm even holding a book (a big one) open, pretending to read it. I look up and say, 'Do you feel tired? Lack the energy you used to have? Get sick often? Then the P-00 Formula probiotic is just the thing for you. Imagine your body as a fertile lawn (I would use the word 'lawn' because it sounds like 'loin', and combined with the word 'fertile', it tends to grab people's attention.) Now let's say weeds start growing on that lawn. You'd want to get rid of them, right? How? Would you use a weed killer and spread toxic chemicals all over your lawn? Or would you want to plant more grass, make the lawn healthier, and *naturally* kill the weed? (Pause for effect. Put the book down. Cross over to a desk with a pill bottle on it.) Your body has *naturally* occurring bacteria inside it. When you get sick, it's because these bacteria are being replaced by illness-causing bugs, just like the weeds on the lawn. Antibiotics are like the chemical weed killer spreading toxins on your lawn. (Pick up a bottle of P-00 Formula. Show label to camera.) A probiotic, like P-00 Formula, *naturally* replaces your body's *natural* bacteria, thus eliminating disease. Try it! If you're not convinced within three months, I will send you a month's supply of your favorite antibiotic absolutely free. Call now.' (Cut to screen with phone number to call and have voice-over rattle off disclaimers very, *very* quickly.)

The probiotic theory is, indeed, an interesting one and it has been proven effective in some cases—specifically in people with diarrhea. The human large intestine does contain a lot of naturally occurring bacteria. An infection in the large intestine, or taking antibiotics, can disrupt the balance and allow abnormal bacteria to grow. This causes diarrhea. Replacing the normal bacteria can help treat the diarrhea. These 'normal' bacteria can be found in various health supplement bottles, but also occur in abundance in yogurt and sauerkraut.

So in order for a probiotic to work, two conditions have to be met: 1) The body part in question must normally have bacteria as a part of it (thus the bladder, kidneys, and lungs are out, to name a few) and 2) the probiotic must be placed directly at the site of the infection. This makes it rather tricky for strep throat and vaginal yeast infections.

In other words, taking a probiotic pill for a cold or a vaginal infection won't help because the probiotic is going into the intestine. It's the same as trying to fix a leaky kitchen sink by spackling the bedroom wall.

So if you ever find yourself in the market for a probiotic, first consider what the problem is that needs treating. If it's anything besides diarrhea, the money would be better spent elsewhere. If it's for diarrhea, consider walking over to the dairy aisle and getting some yogurt. (Unless you're a sauerkraut lover, in which case, you're on your own. As far as I'm concerned it's in the same aisle as Albatross food.) Not only will you get the probiotic, but you'll also get some extra calcium and various vitamins at no extra charge!

Prom Night Blues

There's a buzz of energy in town around June. Adolescents are more restless than usual. Back when I was a senior in high school, circa 1784 CE, we called it 'senioritis'. I'm not sure what it's called these days because I'm old and out of touch. But what I'm fairly certain has not changed is the excitement surrounding graduation, or 'commencement'. Graduation is called 'commencement' because it symbolizes the start of a new phase in life (unless the student is graduating from Donald Trump High School in which case it would be called 'termination'. The graduation ceremony would be very simple: The students stand before the Don. He looks at them and says, 'You're fired!' But I digress.)

An integral part of high school graduation is prom night. The last hurrah for the graduating seniors. A night that is filled with promise, romance, heartbreak, high fashion, and the inevitable pimple.

Like a bad commercial for acne cream, or a cliché movie scene, pimples have a tendency to strike at the most inopportune times. They stand up brazenly and stare back from the mirror with that self-satisfied, life-ruining look.

But why would teenagers get afflicted with acne more than other people? It's not fair! Perhaps Mother Nature feels that school work, a hair-sprouting body, non-understanding parents, and the relentless pursuit of acceptance by one's peers is simply not enough pressure for the typical teenager.

Medically speaking, the raging hormones of teen years have something to do with it. Dietarily speaking, chocolate and fried foods do not—which is unfortunate considering that it has been an effective tool in helping some teens eat better.

Acne is caused by an infection in the oil-producing glands of the skin. Bacteria that normally live on the skin in peace and harmony with the body find their way into these glands. Skin and dirt cover the gland shut and the bacteria start to replicate. And when bacteria replicate, they really trash the place.

The body's immune system rushes in to kick them out. Naturally, the bacteria don't want to leave such a warm, cozy, environment where food is so readily available. The immune cells warn the bacteria, 'Don't make us come in there!' The bacteria reply, 'Oh yeah? You and what army?' A battle thus ensues between the body's infection-fighting cells and the bacteria. The result is redness, swelling, and pus at the gland, resulting in a pimple. Brownheads, blondheads, and redheads are all susceptible to getting blackheads and whiteheads.

Since acne is caused by an infection, washing the skin can help. Using soap specifically designed for acne works best.

There are creams available, too. Advertisements for these creams show a cartoon pimple melting away like the wicked witch in 'The Wizard of Oz' with the application of their product. But keep in mind that particular footage is sped up 648,000 times—meaning that a process which normally takes at least a month is reduced to four seconds.

So what is a teen in a pinch to do when Mount Vesuvius decides to erupt on one's forehead on prom night? For starters, grab a roll of gauze and wrap up both hands like the mummy to prevent the urge to pop it. Yes, it's mouth-wateringly tempting. There's nothing quite like the satisfaction of eviscerating an unruly blemish, even if it does hurt like the dickens. But popping a pimple forces the pus deeper into the skin (even though some of it comes out the top). This makes the infection worse and can cause scarring.

The only viable option on prom night to deal with a pimple is make-up. Ask your mother, girlfriend (female friend or sweetheart), or brother who's into 80's glam rock for a shade that would look most natural, and get spackling!

So enjoy this momentous milestone. The world is your oyster. Wash it down with fries and a chocolate shake. It won't cause acne. But *do* remember to wash your face twice a day. And let the celebrations commence!

The Proof is in the Evidence-Based Pudding

I remember reading in a grade school science text book that each scientific experiment raises more questions than it answers. That was discouraging since it dashed my young hopes of finding an answer to everything. Fortunately, I found out the answer to everything when I turned fourteen without having to bother with 'science' and 'evidence'. And yet, somehow, I forgot it all by the time I graduated college. I should have made notes.

Now I find myself wanting to answer questions that previous articles bring up. In a previous chapter, I talked about the 'Patient-Centered Medical Home' and the term 'evidence-based medicine' came up. So now I feel propelled to clarify.

'Evidence-based medicine', as the name suggests, means using scientific evidence to guide medical decisions. While this may seem obvious, it hasn't always been the case in medicine. For example, the treatment for intestinal tapeworms used to be starvation and placement of a bowl of milk near the patient's mouth. The reasoning was that the tapeworm would get hungry and be lured up to the mouth by the milk. While that seems to make good logical sense, there's no scientific evidence that it works.

In some cultures, people who have diarrhea are deprived of liquids. The reasoning is that since the body is clearly rejecting liquids, it must have a surplus. But scientific evidence has shown that not only will that treatment not work, it will actually make the patient more ill.

In order to establish an 'evidence-based' practice, there has to be good research supporting the practice. For starters, the research must have been done on a large number of people. Let's say I wanted to find out what percentage of the population is left-handed. I could head out into the street, brandishing a clipboard and a retractable pen, grab three people at random and yell, 'You're left-handed, aren't you?' and repeat the phrase while blocking their path until they've answered 'Yes!' Then I could conclude (from the comfort of my mental health residential facility) that 100 percent of the population is left-handed. That conclusion would not expedite my release because the research was done with only three subjects and anyone who draws conclusions on such small numbers clearly should not be let out into society. If I had done the experiment by calmly asking 10,000 people their handedness, then the results would be more reliable. (And I would not have to endure the endless green Jell-O at the mental facility.)

Another criterion that defines good research is how it's designed or carried out. The 'gold-standard' that makes scientific mouths water is a double-blind, randomized, placebo-controlled trial (RCT). If you're ever looking to excite a scientist, simply whisper those words into his/her ear. But be forewarned: they may not be held responsible for their behavior afterwards!

If I were to do research on people's reactions to perceived unstable behavior, I would hire interviewers to go out into public. Half of them would brandish stationery and yell, and the other half would simply ask people in a calm manner their handedness. This would be the placebo-controlled part. I would send interviewers to various locations and make sure they interview people of all races, genders, religions, and body types equally. This would be the 'randomized' part. I would also *not* tell the interviewers or the interviewees what I was looking for. That would be the 'double-blind' part. Then I would publish my results in a prestigious scientific publication and wait for the Nobel Prize to come knocking at my door and pretend not to be home just to watch it squirm.

The third defining quality of good research is that it's reproducible, meaning that other people can carry out the same experiment and get the same results.

Once those criteria are met, then we have an 'evidence-based' practice. And we parade it around town on a float as confetti pours down from skyscrapers. The mayor would give it the key to the city and the 'evidence-based' practice would deliver a speech loaded with feigned humility.

So by using 'evidence-based' practices, we can be assured that we are providing care based on the best information possible. This is not to say that one cannot use the old methods, so long as they cause no harm. If someone chooses to wear a wreath of garlic to ward off the flu, so be it, but I would still recommend they get a flu shot.

The Refined Blood Sucker

After a recent trip to the great Midwest to visit my old stomping grounds, (i.e., the inside of my dingy apartment and the medical school library), I was reminded of all the things I used to associate with the Midwest: large open fields, lush vegetation, exceedingly friendly people (to the point of suspicion), and mosquitoes. Big, hungry, aggressive, prehistoric mosquitoes that can take down a grown buffalo in full flight.

The mosquito has rightfully earned its reputation as one of our most annoying pests by refining its blood-sucking capabilities with a ferocity and attention to detail that would make German car engineers jealous.

Let's look at some of the failed models.

Version1.0: This prototype was large, difficult to maneuver, and landed roughly, alerting its victim to its presence far too easily. It stung as soon as it landed which meant that, more often than not, it didn't even hit a blood vessel. Also, the sting from its nose piercing its victim's skin caused many models to become squashed.

Version 2.0: This model came equipped with a blood sensor in the nose which increased its blood-vessel-hitting capabilities. It had better handling and landed lightly which decreased the victim's awareness of its presence. It came in metallic gray and cobalt blue. Airbags were optional. It was somewhat more successful, but its piercing of the skin still stung, rendering it most inefficient.

Version 2.5: A breakthrough! A reservoir of numbing medication was added to the nose. This version would not only find a blood vessel, but numb the skin before piercing. The victims would hardly notice anything happening. The lightness and maneuverability continued to improve. This version saw the introduction of the eight-speaker Bose sound system. But in beta testing, a lot of the models were coming back empty, with clogged noses. The blood was clotting in the nose before it could be swallowed.

Back to the drawing board.

Then, around 100,000,000 BCE, in the heart of Pangaea, a group of engineers came up with a simple and elegant solution: equip the models with a blood thinner! This kept the blood from clotting and allowed the mosquito to fill its reservoir. This model, called M0sQu/t.0, was a hit. It was lighter and quieter than ever, the sound system was now standard, and it was priced to move. Soon blood was being sucked out of animals all over the world.

The M0sQu/t.0 model, to this day, is the best-selling mosquito version worldwide. It boasts an unrivaled sucking success rate. And with a 2.9 percent APR, and five-year 50,000 suck warranty, it's still hard to resist.

This has led to it becoming the carrier of choice for many diseases, such as malaria and West Nile Virus.

This model, however, still has its flaws. Namely, it makes the victims itch. The mosquito saliva which now numbs the skin and thins the blood also triggers an allergic reaction in the host. The result is swelling, redness and itching at the site of stinging. Unfortunately, once stung, there isn't much the victim can do to stop the itching. Antihistamines, like loratadine (Claritin) and diphenhydramine (Benadryl), are moderately helpful. Calamine lotion helps very little. And contrary to many old wives' tales, pressing a fingernail into the spot to form an X helps only until the pain wears off.

Humans, becoming fed up with itching and catching nasty diseases, have decided to fight back. They've developed creams and sprays that repel the mosquito. They also know to avoid being outside at dusk and dawn when mosquitoes are most active. Some take garlic pills which also repels mosquitoes (with the minor side effect—or benefit—of repelling other humans).

In the United States, disease-carrying mosquitoes are quite rare. But in other parts of the world, protection from mosquitoes is a must. The Center for Disease Control's website, *www.cdc.gov*, has good information regarding mosquito protection and the parts of the world in which it would be needed.

Hopefully, the mosquito engineers will realize that itching and catching illnesses have greatly hindered the success of the mosquito and has caused it to lose market share to the more aesthetic lady bugs and butterflies. Perhaps in the 200,008 model, we will see a friendlier, less illness-causing, and less itch-inducing mosquito.

Refined Grains in Whole Grain Clothing

The silence is broken by the crunch of a Styrofoam cup on the ground, which seems all too happy to be rid of its contents. All heads turn towards the sound. Standing by the window, Pasta pulls back the curtains and a blinding light fills the room. One by one, Breads and Cereals stand up and, shielding their eyes, stammer towards the light. This is unlike any of their previous support group meetings.

Looking out the window, they see a grassy knoll, the man-made lake on the community college grounds, and in the sky, shining brighter than anything they had ever seen before, 'Whole Grains'.

Broad smiles blossom on their faces as they start jumping, yelling and hugging each other. This is it! This is their ticket back to the big life! No longer will they have to justify their existence. No longer will they be seen as an 'addiction.' They can now *be* the healthy choice thanks to the USDA's recommendation that people eat more 'whole grains' as part of a healthy diet.

And before the 'Whole Grains' set that day, they had all re-packaged their products with the words 'whole grains' emblazoned on the packaging. 'Whole Grains' became the new 'extreme' complete with 'Whole Grain Sports' and 'Whole Grain Four Blade Disposable Razors'.

So how did a group of foods go from being the cause of everything from obesity to Alzheimer's to flat hair to being the cure for obesity, Alzheimer's, and split ends?

The answer is in the packaging. Looking closely at the packages of many of these cereal and bread items, one can see that the words 'Whole Grains' are in large font, and in smaller font, in front of the 'Whole Grains', are words like 'Contains . . .' or 'A good source of . . .' or 'Made with . . . .'

Looking on the ingredients list gives us another clue. The first few ingredients are still processed flour and high fructose corn syrup. But further down the order, we see some type of whole grain. In other words, the manufacturer kept the same obesity-inducing, memory-losing, end-splitting recipe and tossed in some whole grains somewhere along the way.

In that spirit, we can all make our own 'Contains Whole Grains' meals at home. Get some pasta, some white bread, and some white rice, put them on a plate and top it with two grains of oatmeal, and voila! A meal 'made with Whole Grains'.

So how is the average consumer to know where the true whole grains lie? That's where the 'Whole Grains Council' comes in. The Whole Grains Council is a group of very regular Jedi Knights who have formed a non-profit consumer advocacy group and are constantly searching for 'chosen' food items that will bring balance to whole grains. When they find one, they put their seal on it. The seal looks like a postage stamp with a wheat plant on it and in the right margin is written 'wholegrainscouncil.org'. The seal can be seen in its entirety on their web site at *www.wholegrainscouncil.org*.

Another way to tell if an item has enough whole grains to do what they're supposed to do is to simply look at the ingredient list. If the very first ingredient is a whole grain, i.e., whole wheat, whole grain rice, whole grain corn, etc., it has enough whole grains to improve health.

So the next time we're looking to do the right thing in the grocery store, let's not be fooled by the words 'Whole Grains' on the package. Let's read the ingredients, and seek out the stamp of the Whole Grains Council. That way we can ensure that we are doing the right thing for our bodies and, most importantly, keeping the USDA happy.

May the whole grains be with us.

(And now, play the drinking game! Read the article again and drink every time you see the phrase 'whole grains'. And don't forget the 'whole grains' mentioned here.)

Rods and Cones

Christmas is a great time of year! Despite a multitude of threats from Grinches and people who don't believe in Santa, Christmas always triumphs! Santa comes to visit all of us who have been good (effectively skipping the gubernatorial mansion in Illinois). Wisely, he flies at night with no lights (unless it's foggy) so as to go undetected. He realizes that while our cones are looking at all the colors on display, our rods will pick up light in our peripheral vision. (Apparently, while the elves pursue dentistry in the off-season, Santa dabbles in ophthalmology.)

Allow me to elaborate: It goes without saying that we use our eyes to see. But more specifically, we use the back part of our eyeball, called the retina, to truly see. In medical school, they told us to think of the retina as the film of a camera. These days, to make it relevant, think of it as the pixels that make up a digital camera. Either way, the image is projected onto the film/pixels, like a projector on a movie screen, and that allows us to see.

Our retina is made up of tiny cells called rods and cones all huddled together like a sea of humanity at a presidential acceptance speech on a cold Chicago night. But this ophthalmologic president still has a long way to go to desegregate the eye. The cones all huddle together in the 'special' spot of the retina where the image is focused most intensely. Cones help us see images and colors clearly.

The rods have to crowd around this 'special' spot and peer over each other's heads just to catch a glimpse of what the eye is looking at. It doesn't help that the cones all giggle and talk amongst themselves about the images. When the rods ask what's going on, the cones reply, 'Oh, nothing.'

I like to think that these rods and cones were named after the famed German physician, Dr. Roderick Kohn, who first discovered these cells and even, though they looked more like rhombuses and trapezoids, he insisted they be called Rods and Kohns (which later became Cones). But the truth is that these cells were named as such because the rods look like rods and the cones look like . . . well . . . cones!

Even though the rods are outside this 'special' area of focus in the retina, they have their own special talent. The rods help us with our peripheral vision and are useful in distinguishing light from dark. So in low lighting, where the cones have a hard time distinguishing color, the rods are called into action. In other words, Christmas time is when the rods sit back and enjoy all the little lights we pick up on our peripheral vision and thus don't feel so deprived.

This is a great time of year to experience this disparity in retinal cell function first hand. On one of those long December nights, try gazing at a faint star. What you will find is that the more you try to focus on it, the dimmer the star gets, but if you look just to the side of the star, suddenly the star appears to brighten. That's the rods picking up the light where the cones could not. Take a moment to allow the rods to relish.

So as we celebrate the holiday season, let's not forget those hard-working rods in our retinas that are kicking it into high gear. Let's take some time to star gaze and look at Christmas lights, if not for the pure fun of it, then just as a way to acknowledge our rods, given that we can't send them Christmas cards. If we did, the cones would have to read it for them.

As for Santa, he might want to reconsider the white trim on his coat. The right moonbeam at the right angle, and all could be lost—for *real* this time!

Say, Say, Say Screening

If I were to make a modernized version of the Paul McCartney and Michael Jackson video for 'Say, Say, Say', I would have them going from town to town in a mobile trailer offering screenings for stroke, peripheral arterial disease (PAD), and abdominal aortic aneurysm (AAA).

For those who don't recall the 80s (willingly or otherwise), the video featured Paul McCartney and Michael Jackson going from town to town selling bottles of a potion that had invigorating properties. Paul would call Michael out of the crowd, have him drink a bottle, and beat their muscular driver at arm wrestling. The townspeople would then storm the wagon, waving money. (Michael Jackson's love interest in the video was played by none other than his sister LaToya. Looking back now, I suppose we should have suspected something even then. But then again, those were the 'Thriller' days. We didn't want to know the truth. But I digress.)

For those of you growing up in the 90s, Paul McCartney was our Jay-Z and Michael Jackson was our Justin Timberlake.

In my modern version of the video, Paul McCartney would distribute fliers around town advertising his services for the nominal fee of—say, say, say—$129. He would have a picture of Michael Jackson smiling in a side bar with a testimonial by him saying that the screening saved his life. They would make sure to target seniors because they tend to be more concerned about their health than the local Brownie Troop.

Paul and Michael would run their tests, produce fancy printed reports complete with neat looking graphics, have it signed off by a Medical Doctor, and move on to the next town.

As they were packing up and counting their money, I'd have Michael Moore burst in on them. He would go up to Paul McCartney, mic in hand, and say, 'Hi, Michael Moore here. So you guys are doing health screenings? It must be very helpful to these people.' Paul McCartney would try to answer, but Michael

Moore would press on, 'So, tell me about the research that's been done that shows that people who get your screenings live longer and stay healthier than people who don't.'

This is where Michael Jackson would spring into action. He would get up and say, 'Before I had my screening, I couldn't do this.' He would proceed to do the splits, come up, turn around and do the moonwalk. Michael Moore would interrupt, 'But this is a testimonial. Tell me about the research'.

Then Michael Moore's voice-over would say, 'Actually, there was no research. There is no evidence that these screenings help people live better or longer. Getting blood pressure under control and having regular health checkups does far more than any of these 'screenings'.' (He would be very careful not to mention anything about weight loss.)

The problem that Michael Jackson and Paul McCartney ran into in my modern remake of the video was that they tried to sell their scheme as a legitimate health-saving tool. They marketed it to people who weren't having any symptoms, which is one of the hallmarks of a screening test. However, in order for a test to truly be a screening test, other criteria must be met. Performing the test must prevent complications of an illness and help people live longer and better. (Mammograms, colonoscopies, and cholesterol checks are examples of good screening tests.) The mobile trailer tests have not been shown to do that.

Furthermore, if one of these tests comes out abnormal, the patient's healthcare provider would have to repeat the test to confirm the findings.

This is why health insurance companies, who normally cover a wide variety of screening tests, do not cover Paul McCartney and Michael Jackson's tests.

Perhaps Paul and Michael would be better off sticking with the invigorating formulas. Although, I would definitely suggest a different love interest. I wonder if Justin Timberlake's sister is busy . . . .

(*Editor's Note*: This was written before the untimely death of Michael Jackson, and is dedicated to his memory.)

Scaling Down (Dandruff)

What's on the mind of dandruff sufferers? Literally, it would be dandruff. Figuratively, it is dandruff as well. This double-mind occupation can be a great opportunity for very efficient mindfulness. But in such an intense state of mindfulness, one would see that dandruff is but a scaly expression of the perfection of life. The falling scales represent the shedding of the old to make way for the new. This would then take dandruff off the mind (figuratively) and break the mindful state, which would then put dandruff back on the mind again. And thus we have one of the few mental vicious cycles that can be broken with a medicated shampoo.

Dandruff is one of the few scalp-related medical conditions that has become immortalized in film by Ally Sheedy's character in 'The Breakfast Club' who made it 'snow' on a picture she drew. I went for days expressing my disgust to anyone and everyone who would listen to make sure no one suspected me of doing such an act. (And yet, one cannot deny the deviant satisfaction of so easily adding texture to a drawing.) But I digress.

Dandruff is a condition in which the scalp gets itchy and starts to flake off. Since dry skin also flakes off, many people think that dandruff is caused by over-washing the hair. Nothing could be further from the truth—except stating that I'm glad I don't own a third generation iPhone. Sure, it tilts and swings and shakes and flashes (the iPhone, not the dandruff), but I've heard it is ergonomically unsound. Now . . . where was I?

Not only is dandruff not caused by over-washing the hair, but washing the hair and scalp regularly can help prevent and possibly treat dandruff.

Dandruff is caused by a fungus. Yes, the good organisms that brought us ringworm, athlete's foot, and a rhyme for 'among us' did not neglect our scalps. Once the fungus gets on the scalp, it starts to cause inflammation which brings about the redness, the itching and the flaking. People with dandruff might become self-conscious about their condition, causing them to skip social events without prior notice. This can then cause others to label them a 'flake' which would further exacerbate their social isolation since they would think people are commenting on their dandruff and not their neglect of social events. This stream of misunderstandings could (if one is desperate enough) lay the foundation for a really bad sitcom entitled 'The Flakey Flake' about a man with dandruff who skips social events. He would, ironically, breakfast on Cheerios because he has a cholesterol problem, too. The series would end with him purchasing dandruff shampoo.

But I digress . . . again . . .

Since dandruff is caused by a fungus, anti-fungal medications can help clear it. There are many over-the-counter medicated shampoos available. They are most effective when used daily, and most importantly, they should be left on for long enough. The lathered shampoo should stay in contact with the scalp for at least five minutes to allow the fungus-killing medication to do its fungus killing.

If over-the-counter shampoos don't work, prescription shampoos are available. These shampoos are applied twice a week in the same manner mentioned above. One can use over-the-counter dandruff shampoos the other days of the week for an added fungus-killing boost.

So for those readers out there who have been disturbed enough by this article to want to *prevent* dandruff, consider washing your hair regularly—ideally, everyday. If dandruff should occur, know that there are plenty of treatment options available. A trip to your local drug store or a consultation with your primary care provider can get things going in the right direction.

But you might want to finish that drawing first.

Serotonin It Down

With the stock market in freefall and Thanksgiving looming, many people have serotonin on (or off) their minds.

Serotonin is a neurotransmitter. Its job is to help nerve cells in the brain communicate with each other. Since communication is the key to a healthy relationship, serotonin plays a very important part in keeping brain cells happy. Here's how it works: Let's suppose that Harry, the brain cell, is trying to say something to Sally, the brain cell. (Maybe he wants to compliment her on how trim her axon looks—has she lost weight?) Harry would release a bunch of serotonin towards Sally, but in order not to overwhelm Sally and seem desperate, Harry immediately starts to suck the serotonin back in! It may not be the most efficient way of doing things, but that's how it is in the brain. (And the DMV.)

When serotonin levels get low in the brain, people can experience depression. Or when people get depression, their serotonin levels drop. It's unclear which causes which. Whenever we ask who started it, they simply point at each other. Either way, increasing serotonin in the brain can help ease the symptoms of depression.

To that end, we have the Selective Serotonin Reuptake Inhibitors (SSRIs).

These medications were a breakthrough when they broke onto the scene twenty-some years ago. They worked well and had surprisingly few side effects. (Don't tell Tom Cruise I said that.) Up until that point, the medications used for depression sometimes caused more problems than they cured.

As the name suggests, these medications block the reuptake of serotonin by brain cells. In other words, when Harry releases serotonin towards Sally, an SSRI will prevent Harry from sucking back his own serotonin, thus leaving more serotonin for Sally to see. Sally, seeing the exuberance of Harry, gets a lift and smiles.

There are many medications in the SSRI family: fluoxetine (Prozac), paroxetine (Paxil), and sertraline (Zoloft) to name a few. But they all do the same thing: increase serotonin. So the stock broker who has felt his serotonin plunge with the DOW can benefit from taking an SSRI.

Serotonin has also been blamed for the drowsy feeling after having a turkey dinner. The reasoning here is that turkey has tryptophan, which is a building block for serotonin. When someone eats a lot of tryptophan, the body must turn it into a lot of serotonin and the consumer becomes sleepy.

That is untrue. It is a negative attack by the Association of Turkey Eating and Living Large (ATE aLL) to prevent people from being concerned about their post-turkey-dinner somnolence. If one were to consume the amount of fat and calories in a typical Thanksgiving meal, without turkey, one would still get equally sleepy. Alternatively, for those willing to brave family wrath, try having some turkey this Thanksgiving *without* gravy or any other sides except salad. Wash it down with plain water, and see how you feel. You'll be painting eyeballs on eyelids and dipping napping family members' hands in warm water all afternoon. Another blow against the ATE aLL's misrepresentation is that people with depression still have depression after turkey dinner.

What the ATE aLL didn't realize is that by this smear on serotonin, it has also driven away its long-time constituent, the brain's sleep center. In a recent press conference, the sleep center decried that serotonin is not the only thing that controls people's sleep cycles. If that were so, then all the people taking SSRIs would be sleeping their lives away. While some SSRIs can cause drowsiness, the majority don't.

So chin up, America! I hear the economy will recover within seven years. In the meantime, perhaps having less turkey this Thanksgiving will be better for our budget. And having less of everything else will be better for our overall alertness.

Show No MRSA

As we walk down the hall of worrisome medical topics, we stroll past the Ebola virus. The movie 'Outbreak' is playing in the background featuring Dustin Hoffman, Renee Russo, and a certain other actor who is currently the star of a wildly successful medically-themed TV show. (Let's just say he followed his 'McDreamy' all the way to the little screen.)

Further down is West Nile and SARS, both adorned with far eastern silk and very large, intricately decorated vases. Seeing a crowd ahead, we move in closer to take a look at the most recent exhibit: MRSA—full name, Methicillin Resistant Staphylococcus Aureus. This is the hot new thing. (Avian flu is sooo behind us.) The exhibit looks like a dirty kitchen. Underneath the scientific name, we see its nickname, 'The bacterial cockroach'.

That is how a prominent physician with the Center for Disease Control (CDC) has described MRSA. When it comes to naming illnesses, the CDC is the Coco Chanel of the Infectious Disease world. Everyone else simply hails their genius and falls in line.

Here is what I believe the CDC is trying to convey with that analogy: 1) MRSA has been around for a while; 2) it acts like a pest, meaning that it can make people ill, but its presence doesn't imply imminent death; and 3) some simple hygiene measures can help control it. (I wonder if this means that it would survive a nuclear fallout as well.)

There are many different kinds of Staphylococcus bacteria. Those who get tired of saying (or typing) Staphylococcus call it Staph—as in 'Let's have a staff meeting to discuss the staff who have Staph".

All humans have Staph on their skin. It's called Staph Epidermidis and it's a relative of Staph Aureus.

Staph Aureus can also live on human skin, but not in terribly large amounts. Sometimes it hides in the nose. Most of the time, it simply sits on the skin looking around at its Staph Epi cousins and asks repeatedly, 'Hey, whatcha doin'?' (The Staph Epis do not typically respond, except for the occasional condescending look.)

But sometimes, when there are tiny breaks in the skin, Staph Aureus decides to go under the skin. Once there, it causes an infection. The patient experiences red bumps, boils or abscesses (pus pockets). Most of the time, they go away with or without antibiotics.

Much like the little girl who breaks the cookie jar, hands her little brother the last cookie and runs away just as mom and dad arrive on the scene, Staph Aureus has an uncanny way of making people believe that they've received a 'spider bite.' Speaking on behalf of my arachnid brethren, nothing could be further from the truth. Spiders rarely bite people. (Unless you're a school photographer and the spider is radioactive.) In fact, I think now is an appropriate time to give a shout out to all my eight-legged homies for keeping the peace and continuing to rid us of other pesky insects in spite of all these false accusations. But I digress.

MRSA is regular Staph Aureus that has become resistant to multiple antibiotics. Those most at risk for getting MRSA used to be people who were hospitalized and/or had a weakened immune system. But lately, it has started to show up in healthy people as well.

Even so, most people with MRSA infections who are otherwise healthy recover without incident. Serious infections from MRSA are still quite rare in this population.

MRSA can spread from person to person either through direct contact or through contaminated personal items like towels, sheets, razor blades, etc. Like most infectious diseases, regular washing with soap and water can help prevent the spread of this illness. Also, using antibiotics judiciously can help prevent the development of more resistant bacteria.

So this holiday season, let's exercise caution when using antibiotics to treat colds. Let's wash our hands and personal items regularly. By this time next year, hopefully we can stroll right past the food crumbs around the MRSA exhibit and on to the hot new worrisome medical topic—whatever it may be. Perhaps it'll be Canada's turn to contribute. One can only hope.

Signs of Sinusitis

Every year when the cold and flu season is in full swing, I'm sure some cold sufferers out there are thinking that they need another sinus infection like they need another hole in their heads. Perhaps they might find irony in the fact that the sinuses are, indeed, holes in the head. (If they don't find it ironic, then I hope that they'd at least find it kind of funny in an interesting, if not a 'ha ha', way.)

We have four major sinuses in the face: one underneath each eye, and one above each eyebrow. There are a lot of theories as to why we have these sinuses. Some believe they act as a barrier—a moat of sorts—between the outside world and the brain. I can see why some would believe that, since our brains are dangerously close to the nasty, bug-ridden outside world. Thanks to our ears, noses, and mouths, each of these can become a virtual microbial highway to the brain.

Others believe that we have sinuses to resonate our voices. Much the same way that the hollow part inside a guitar or violin helps to amplify the sound, our sinuses help amplify our voices. Imagine the sinuses like showers. Everyone sounds like Andrea Bocelli and/or Christina Aguilera when they sing in the shower because the sound resonates off the walls. The sinuses accomplish the same thing but in a much more portable way—like a zero-bedroom, four-bath luxury town home embedded in the face. The location's great, although the view leaves something to be desired. Also, it gets rather drafty at times.

Regardless of theories of origin, sinuses have been a cause of discomfort for many years. In fact, all evidence to the contrary, I believe that the ancient inhabitants of Mesopotamia were so bothered by their sinuses that they decided to name a mountain in honor of their troubles, using the ancient plural form of sinus, Sinai. Perhaps this is why so many hospitals are named after it.

Our sinuses cause discomfort when they become infected. This can happen after a cold or a flare-up of allergies. The sinuses get filled with mucus, and bacteria grow. As more and more mucus accumulates, one feels pain and pressure where the sinuses are (below the eyes and/or above the eyes), and a green river comes streaming from the nose, not unlike the Tigris and Euphrates which, incidentally, are both right next to Mount Sinai. Some people feel pain in their upper teeth which are the downstairs neighbors of the sinuses. The pain and pressure worsen when one leans forward.

Just like any plugged-up cavity, draining the cavity can help release pressure and, in the case of the sinuses, bring relief of symptoms. This can be done with a decongestant. These days, there are two main decongestants available over the counter: pseudoephedrine (Sudafed) and phenylephrine (Neo-Synephrine). Although they are both available without a prescription, pseudoephedrine is kept behind the counter. All one has to do is ask for it, sign a paper, give a driver's license, get fingerprinted, have a retinal scan, and leave a blood and urine sample. This heightened security is thanks to some people who have figured out how to make methamphetamines out of pseudoephedrine.

When decongestants fail to cure a sinus infection, or do not help the symptoms, antibiotics may be warranted.

So the next time Mount Sinai erupts and the banks of the Tigris and Euphrates are flooded with green mucus, it could be the sinuses getting infected. Consider a decongestant if your healthcare provider thinks it's appropriate. And let's keep our facially embedded showers slime free so that we may sing an ode to our uninfected brains.

Singing Mammogram

I think a singing mammogram would be a much better way to remind women that they are due for their annual breast cancer screening than a card or a phone call. Of course the singer would have to be lying on a large, flat piece of metal with a second large, flat piece right on top of him or her. It might not be the ideal conditions for a singer, but neither is American Idol and look how well they've fared.

Much like how the rate of women dying from cervical cancer dramatically decreased with the advent of the Pap smear, the rate of women dying from breast cancer has dramatically decreased since the invention of the mammogram.

Yes, Mr. Mammo's ingenious idea of taking X-rays of breasts to check for early cancerous lesions proved to be quite a breakthrough. Most people have seen videos or pictures of women getting mammograms on various news reports. The shot is always from behind, carefully angled to convey what is happening without being overly revealing. The lighting is soft and the camera lens is ever so slightly out of focus, much like those movie adaptations of Jane Austen novels.

So who qualifies for this wonderful service? The answer is quite all-encompassing: any woman over 40. But wait! You 35 to 39.9-year-olds won't get off the hook that easily. It is recommended that you have one at anytime during those years. This is known as the 'baseline'. Sort of a radiographic 'before' shot to which all the 'after' 40 shots will be compared. Some of those after-40 mammograms go on to develop complexes after being constantly compared to the more youthful, and dense, 35-to-39.9-year-old mammograms. But after years of therapy and many self-help books, they learn to love themselves for the beautiful mammograms they are. They learn to take pride in their more translucent appearance, which is more conducive to detecting breast cancer anyway.

A mammogram is performed by placing the breast on a flat piece of metal, and placing a second flat piece on top of it. The two plates are tightened to make the breast as flat as possible. Then X-rays are taken at different angles. Radiologists look at the X-rays for suspicious spots. Some women have described it as a 'boob sandwich with breads of steel.' (I can see why!)

Although mammograms have been proven effective in their own right, they do have their shortcomings. They can miss about 10 percent of suspicious spots. That's where the healthcare provider comes in. By doing a breast exam in the office, he/she can check for the spots that a mammogram can miss. The two are the dynamic duo in the fight against breast cancer. I like to think of healthcare providers as Batman and mammograms as Robin—and not just because of Batman's more stylish outfit. Perhaps we could have a national contest to come up with other superhero analogies like Spot-Seeker and Miss Mash, or Sensor and Zappor. The winner would then launch a series of comic books designed to educate young people on the importance of screening for breast cancer. But I digress.

It's a good idea to have the breast exam before the mammogram. That way, if there is a suspicious spot on the exam, the healthcare provider (aka Batman) can send a note to the mammographer to focus in on that area.

If there is a suspicious spot on the mammogram, sometimes women have to go back for a repeat mammogram with 'magnified' views of the area. This helps to determine what the appropriate next step would be, i.e., a repeat mammogram in six months or a biopsy.

So, women over 40, mark your calendars and set your alarms. Everyone else, send singing telegram/mammograms to your loved ones to remind them to go in for a breast exam and mammogram every year and, together, we can put the squeeze on breast cancer. I'm just glad we don't check for testicular cancer that way.

(*Editor's Note*: This was written before the USPSTF's recommendation against routine mammograms for women 40 to 49, but is still very relevant. See the chapter on 'Clarifamography' for more information.)

Skin Alphabetry

Summer is here! Why, it only seems like 365 days ago when we celebrated the solstice and here we are again! It's like the annual 'Going Out of Business' sale at the local furniture store!

For some people, summertime means showing more skin. For many others, it means seeing more skin. Since we have all this skin on display and so many eyes to observe, I feel this is a great opportunity to get some very important work done: namely, screening for suspicious skin spots.

Thanks to Mother Nature, there's a relatively easy way to remember which skin spots are suspicious and which are less suspicious. They're called the 'ABCDs' of skin spots. As we'll soon see, this definitively proves that Mother Nature speaks English. (How else would one explain apple, lettuce and thyme all having English names?)

To make it even easier to remember, we can make a song and sing it to the tune of L-O-V-E by Nat King Cole. It's a very famous song that everyone knows—even people who've never heard it. But if you need a reminder, any music search engine has it and will play a 30-second clip for free. You always have the option of buying the song for $0.99 and listening to the entire thing—provided there's enough money left over from your government economic stimulus rebate check. But I digress.

So here goes my rendition of 'ABCD of skin spots' sang to the tune of 'L-O-V-E'.

'A is fo-or a-a-symm-etry (stretch the syllables to make it work)/ B is for the border that you see/ C is for the color/ uniform there is no other/ D is for dia-meter/ the smaller it is that's better . . . .' Thank you for coming. You're a beautiful crowd. Try the $3.99 prime rib special.

Now that we have the song stuck in our heads, let's go over what it really means.

A stands for asymmetry. The 'a-' part means 'without', and 'symmetry' means each side is a mirror reflection of the other. For example, Johnny Depp's face is symmetric. If we draw a line down the middle, one side is the mirror reflection of the other. On the other hand, a Picasso rendition of Johnny Depp's face would not be symmetric because both eyes would be on one side and the mouth would be in between them and, on the other side, would be his big toe.

So a skin spot that is symmetric is less suspicious, whereas one that is asymmetric is more suspicious.

B stands for border. If I—er—I mean someone—had a tattoo of Johnny Depp's face, the borders (aka outline) of the tattoo would be smooth, making it a less suspicious lesion. If someone had a tattoo of Keith Richards' face, the border would be jagged and he would be considered a more suspicious lesion.

C stands for color. If the entire lesion is one color, it's less suspicious. If the color varies in different parts of the same lesion, it's more suspicious.

D stands for diameter which means how big it is. If it is greater than six millimeters across, it's more suspicious. For those of you who are not from Canada or Europe or Latin/Central America or Asia or Africa, six millimeters is about a quarter of an inch. (Hopefully, the rest of the world will wake up someday and convert to the American system so we can do away with all this confusion.)

But the most important thing to keep in mind is that these are merely guidelines. If there's any question at all, it's worthwhile to have the lesion examined by a healthcare professional. Also, if a lesion is changing in size, shape, or color, it needs to be evaluated by a healthcare professional regardless of how many 'less suspicious' properties it has.

So let's make the most of our idle time this summer. Whether lounging at the beach, ignoring the safety demonstration on an airplane, or waiting for a pump at the only gas station in town with regular unleaded under $4.00, let's take some time to examine our skin and the skin of our loved ones. It will be time well spent.

The Splinted Shins

If I were giving a speech to the American College of Sports Medicine, I would start with a joke: 'Why were the high school track athletes walking on their heels? Because they were trying to heal their shin splints!' The audience would erupt in boisterous laughter and deep inside I would cry a little because that really is what I did in high school. Back then I was just a soccer player in short-shorts and spikes. I did as I was told.

Of course, in those days, my high school had the unforgiving black asphalt track. Nowadays, it's the all-weather ground rubber surface that gives foot massages and back therapy. Kids, these days!

My understanding of shin splints is different now (and hopefully more accurate). Shin splints are an 'overuse injury'. This means that there are no heroic saves/tackles/runs/dives to explain the injury. This is not to say that one cannot be made up. I wish I had told my friends in high school that I had injured my legs breaking cinder blocks with consecutive jumping round-houses without touching the ground like a Crouching Tiger or a Hidden Dragon. (And thanks to *Facebook.com*, I still can!)

Shin splints tend to occur in runners who have had a change in training, specifically an increase in intensity or distance (by more than 10 percent), or a change in running surface.

Shin splints cause pain along the outer edge of the shin bone. The area becomes sore to the touch. In mild cases, the pain occurs mainly with activity, but in severe cases, it can be present even at rest.

Shin splints are also called 'medial tibial stress syndrome'. In spite of the fancy name, it is actually a poorly understood process. There is evidence that inflammation of muscle and/or the outer covering of the bone are involved. But we haven't been able to pin it down any more accurately than that. In fact, I believe shin splints are what led Heisenberg to his Uncertainty Principle. He initially tried to pin down the exact cause of shin splints. The more he tried to pin down the location, the less accurate the measurement of inflammation. From there it was a simple extrapolation to electrons. But I digress.

The treatment of shin splints is the same as any other overuse injury.

'Relative rest' is key. This means cutting back activity to a level that is comfortable. Sometimes it means not running for seven to ten days, then gradually resuming. If it is imperative that one exercise to keep up endurance, bicycling, swimming, water running, and elliptical training are acceptable forms of exercise until the pain resolves. Then activities should be resumed starting with low intensity and short duration, and gradually increasing.

Anti-inflammatories like ibuprofen (Advil, Motrin) or naproxen (Aleve) taken regularly for two weeks can also help. For people with 'flat feet' or high arches, inserts or orthotics might help.

Many other modalities, such as ice, ultrasound, stretching, acupuncture, aroma therapy and exorcism, have been tried and none have been found to be superior to relative rest and anti-inflammatories. Ironically, splinting has never been an option.

One important distinction to be made from shin splints is a tibial (aka shin bone) stress fracture. A stress fracture is a very small fracture that might not show up on an X-ray. Therefore, if the pain is not improving as expected, it's always wise to see a healthcare professional.

So happy running, everyone! Just remember to increase running distance and intensity slowly, run on softer surfaces, and wear appropriate footwear. If pain does start on the outside edge of the shin bone, try relative rest and anti-inflammatories early in the course. It can mean a speedier recovery. And may all our shins go un-splinted and all our splints go un-shinned.

Spring into Action

Spring is in the air! The signs are all around us: the sun carves a higher arc across the sky, cats in heat make that incredibly human-baby-like sound, and the small print under March 20 on the calendar reads, 'vernal equinox'. An 'equinox' is when the sun passes over the intersection of the ecliptic and celestial equators. We get two of them a year. One marks the beginning of spring and the other the beginning of fall. This is not to be confused with 'Hardnox' which is where all the gold in the country is kept. Naturally, it is heavily fortified. In fact, the name comes from the action needed to get anyone's attention in that place. The place where people get trained to watch over all the gold in the country is called 'the School of Hardnox.'

But I digress.

As the days get longer (thanks in part to the new-and-improved-three-weeks-earlier Daylight Savings Time), people spend more time outdoors admiring nature in bloom, the turning of the seasons, and the rebirth of various animals. But nature also has its naughty side. Yes, it beckons us with fragrances and colors, but pokes us with thorns and makes us itch with poison oak.

Most people know that poison oak has 'leaves of three' and therefore it is wise to 'leave them be' (to which the great philosopher Homer [Simpson] replied, 'Leaves of four, eat some more'). Most people also have their own recipe for dealing with potential exposure to poison oak. Some take a cold shower right afterwards. Some scrub with Ajax. Personally, I like to indulge in a big bowl of chocolate ice cream. After all, if I'm going to itch, I might as well enjoy things while I can.

What makes poison oak 'poisonous' is the oil. When the plant's oil gets on the skin, it starts an allergic reaction. But this is not a typical allergic reaction; it's a 'delayed' one—meaning that the reaction doesn't start until a day or two after exposure. (It's not unlike that incredibly witty comeback one thinks of two days after someone has made a snide remark at a dinner party.)

Some people are more sensitive to this oil than others. There are tales of brave souls who have rolled around in poison oak trying to prove that they're 'immune' to it—which turns out to be a good example of 'famous last words'.

That's where nature is its trickiest: the more someone is exposed to something, the more allergic they can become to that substance. In other words, every repeated exposure to poison oak can bring about a stronger reaction.

Washing the skin as soon as possible after exposure can help minimize the reaction. Once the oil is washed off, it can no longer spread. However, since it is a 'delayed' reaction, new spots can appear over time.

A poison oak rash tends to consist of itchy red lines on the exposed areas of the skin. Sometimes blisters develop. The fluid in these blisters is what the body has made as a result of the allergic reaction. Since the body makes this fluid, it has no poison oak in it and thus is incapable of spreading the rash.

Typically, medical intervention is needed for a poison oak rash to go away. For small patches of relatively mild reaction, a prescription steroid cream can help. For stronger or more widespread reactions, steroid pills can be helpful.

As with most things, 30 ml of prevention is worth 0.45 kg of cure. So wearing long-sleeved shirts and pants, and avoiding contact with suspicious plants is helpful.

So let's enjoy this spectacular display that nature has put on for us. Let's spring like a spring over a spring in spring, all the while keeping a respectable distance from the surrounding foliage. Enjoying nature is like petting a cat: pet the soft furry side, beware the sharp, claw-y side.

(*Author's Note:* Cats in heat should be considered sharp and claw-y all around.)

Stand-Off at the FP, IM, GP Corral

It was high noon at Greenville Hospital. The fluorescent lights were blazing directly overhead as Dr. A and Dr. B squared off in the hallway, their hands suspended at their sides. We were busily scanning their bodies for what they could draw. A prescription pad? Lounge keys? A clicky pen? Someone rolled tumbleweed for effect. But we all agreed the vulture was a bit much.

The residents gathered behind their respective department heads: The Family Practice residents behind Dr. A, and the Internal Medicine residents behind Dr. B.

Internal Medicine had long ruled the wards of the County Hospital, but now Family Practice wanted to start taking care of its own patients when they were hospitalized.

'Why you lily-livered-long-legged-land-lover.' We were all astounded! Dr. A, who was of Indian origin, could drawl! She continued, 'We want to start taking care of our own patients when they get admitted to the hospital, be they adult, child, or pregnant woman, because that is our training. We do three years of it after medical school.'

Now we were stupefied! Dr. A had a gift for exposition!

'Now listen here, you cherry-chompin'-chigger of a cherub', Dr. B shot back, 'We been runnin' this here hospital since my great-great-gran'pappy rode in to town with nothing but his stethoscope, his list of HMO formularies, and his Palm Pilot. (Back then it was called an 'abacus' and tech support was a pair of pliers.) We will tend to every adult admitted and adults only because that's what we Internists do. We are doctors for adults. We, too, do three years of training after we graduate medical school.'

'So wait a minute, are you Internists or interns?'

We all looked around. That sound had not come from either of our department heads. And there, holding the tumbleweed, was a patient.

'An intern is a general term given to anyone who is in their first year of training after medical school. Surgeons, radiologists, anesthesiologists, pediatricians, family physicians and, yes, internists all do an internship and are called 'interns' for that year', came the answer from Dr. B.

'An Internist intern?' asked the patient. That did sound confusing.

The patient turned to us, 'So what about GPs?'

Dr. A fielded this one. 'GP, or General Practitioner, is any doctor who starts working right after medical school without doing a residency. There are fewer and fewer of them these days. Virtually all medical school graduates do some type of residency and those who like the broad scope of General Practice do Family Practice residencies and become Family Physicians.'

'So in other words, an intern can be of any specialty, but is only an intern for a year. An Internist is a primary care doctor for adults. And a Family Physician is a primary care doctor for adults, children and pregnant women' summarized the patient.

'Actually, there is a caveat to that', I chimed in. 'Very few Family Practitioners are providing care for pregnant women these days because of the lifestyle and the malpractice premiums.' Catching Dr. A's disapproving glance, I quickly added, 'But we still enjoy doing it!'

Drs. A and B turned their attention to each other again. Eyes squinting, fingers twitching as they stared and stared. And just then, at the height of the tension, a bell rang. The elevator doors opened and they both stepped inside. 'I hope the cafeteria has grilled chicken sandwiches today', Dr. B said as the door began to close. 'My treat', said Dr. A.

We residents were left standing, mouths agape. They were going to get to the cafeteria before us! Panicked, we ran to the stairwell. Drs. A and B always held up the line chatting with other attendings and we had rounds in half an hour! Darn them and their expositions!

Striking for Health, Health Strikes Back

Is it just me or are there a lot of angry people holding signs outside grocery stores these days? From what little I understand, it seems to have to do with healthcare coverage, or lack thereof.

This is but a tiny bubble in the smoldering cauldron that is the US healthcare delivery system. (I can't wait for the new Harry Potter movie to come out!) As with most things that bring unrest, it has to do with money.

In the United States, we have the best healthcare system in the world. We have the best trained doctors, the latest equipment, the most up-to-date facilities, and many fancy drugs, all of which cost money. Add to that the bureaucratic alphabet soup that needs satiating (i.e., JHACO, HIPAA, PCOT, etc.), and you have a recipe for unaffordable healthcare. The system is great. The *delivery* of healthcare is the problem.

It's becoming harder and harder for any entity—from insurance companies to employers to individuals—to pay for medical care.

The insurance companies tried to control costs with their HMO 'product' which was billed as an all-access pass to Disneyland. Pay a fee and get in to the healthcare park. But soon, we realized that food wasn't included. There were height limits, expectant mothers and people with back problems could not ride, and you couldn't climb the trees.

Now the secret's out. Everybody knows that HMO is cheap insurance. Everybody is also painfully realizing that you get what you pay for, even in healthcare. On the other hand, if it weren't for HMOs, most people wouldn't have *any* health coverage.

I attended an interesting talk by an economist last year. (Never thought I'd say 'economy' and 'interesting' in the same sentence.) He said the trend in healthcare in the years to come will be to shift more cost to the patient. We are already seeing this as co-pays have increased for emergency room visits and non-formulary medications.

In a way, patients now have more choices. You *could* go to the emergency room for a cold sore. You *could* get the latest brand-name medication. But you'll have to pay more.

The government tried to sort out the mess in the 90's when Hillary Clinton gathered the brightest medical and economic minds of the time and spent six months studying the problem. In the end, they all threw their hands up and walked away, leaving the problem to sort itself out.

And things *will* sort themselves out. It's just a matter of time. However, until that happens, there will be many unhappy people who will be uninsured or underinsured. As a patient, be ready to have to pay more.

The irony of it all is that, as a nation, we have spent so much time and effort to make our healthcare second to none, that now we can't even afford it.

The Summer of Itch

Summer pop quiz, people! What is itchy, affects the skin of allergy sufferers, and rhymes with 'exhuma'? No, not 'dermatophytosis'. Guess again! No, not 'lichen simplex chronicus'. Guess again! That's right, eczema! Well done! And for your prize, simply go to the nearest window and open it: it's fresh air! (Not available in all areas. Void where prohibited. Taxes not included.)

So summertime is a time for eczema especially in dry areas like the Southwest and West Coast. But why would it be so? Is it not enough that allergy sufferers have to suffer with itchy eyes, noses, ears, and throats? Have they not suffered enough? Don't answer that. It's a rhetorical question. A rhetorical question is something that has to do with a rhetory. A rhetory is a proposed explanation for something that is not yet scientifically proven, like the rhetory of evolution.

But I digress.

The key to understanding eczema is moisture. By Intelligent Design, the skin of allergy sufferers does not hold moisture as well as the skin of non-allergy sufferers. (Calls to Intelligent Design were not immediately returned.) When the skin becomes dry, it can get inflamed and itchy. It can go on to become thick and flakey. This is called eczema. While eczema can strike anywhere on the body, it's most common on the arms and legs—specifically in front of the elbows and behind the knees.

Since moisture—or lack thereof—is the problem, then the answer must be moisturization. And it is—depending on the method used. Simply getting the skin wet can actually worsen the problem. As the skin dries, either on its own or with a towel, more moisture leaves the skin making the skin drier. Being more active in the summer (and hence needing to bathe more often), or partaking in water activities, winds up exacerbating eczema.

But moisturizing with lotion can help replenish moisture to the skin and reduce the discomfort of eczema. Since no self-respecting man would ever be caught applying lotion, I suggest placing it in a canister labeled 'Sports Cream for Men with Too Many Muscles—Also Cures Leather!'—and watch the women swoon. The same technique can be used by women who are looking for a non-confrontational way to deal with unwanted attention. The best part about using a moisturizer is that it is virtually impossible to overdo it. It's always better to err on moisturizing too often than not often enough.

All this talk about prevention is fine, but what is an allergy sufferer to do when eczema does strike? (This is *not* a rhetorical question. It has been answered scientifically.) That's when the steroid creams come in. Steroids are the ultimate anti-inflammatory medication. Luckily, since eczema is confined to the skin, putting steroid cream on affected areas can reduce inflammation directly where it is needed with virtually no effect on the rest of the body.

Over-the-counter hydrocortisone cream can help for mild cases. For more severe cases of eczema, prescription steroid creams may be needed. A quick trip to your local primary care provider can get you well on your way to the exact same you, except wrapped in healthier, less itchy, and less flakey packaging.

Since steroid creams can take up to two weeks to yield results, anti-histamines, like loratadine, can give more immediate relief whilst in eczema purgatory.

So this summer, as allergy sufferers enjoy the warm weather, may they keep lots of lotion handy, and footy, and body-y, and back-y to prevent eczema. But if eczema does strike, strike back with some intelligently designed steroids. Perhaps a friendly neighbor will share his/her leather-curing salve.

Super Bugs

Wearing microscopic spandex suits and funny masks, 'super bugs' are becoming more and more of a menace to the concerned citizens of planet Earth. What makes them 'super'? Nothing good, that's for sure! Their 'superness' comes from their ability to survive attacks by antibiotics. They've gained their 'super' powers through humans' inappropriate use of antibiotics.

It all started with the discovery of the first antibiotic, penicillin. Until then, bleeding and exorcism were the preferred ways of treating infections. With the discovery of penicillin, all that changed. Soon leeches and exorcists found their jobs outsourced and had to seek vocational rehab (which is extremely difficult for leeches. Sucking blood is pretty much their only gig.)

We humans were drunk with the power of penicillin. We used it to treat many illnesses, regardless of whether or not it was caused by bacteria. Pneumonia? Penicillin. Heartburn? Penicillin! Dyslexia? Penicillin!! After all, what was the harm? We might as well cover all the bases.

We soon noticed, however, that some bacteria refused to die with penicillin. That's when the arms race started. We made antibiotics, the bacteria became resistant, we made new antibiotics to fight the resistant bacteria, and the bacteria became resistant to those as well. And today we find ourselves nearly at the end of the road. There are super bugs out there that only one or two antibiotics can kill. We just have our fingers crossed that they don't become resistant to those one or two antibiotics; otherwise, we have to train new leeches and exorcists.

All the while that humans were engaged in the arms race with bacteria, viruses went about their usual business—they infected people and caused illnesses that had similar symptoms to bacterial infections. Viruses are the group of organisms that bring us the common cold, the flu (respiratory, intestinal, and avian), rabies, SARS, and the more exotic Ebola (remember that one?).

All too often, for various reasons, doctors would treat viral infections with antibiotics. Every time we did so, the bacteria became stronger.

Bacteria and viruses have about as much in common as fleas and ringworm. Both fleas and ringworm can cause an itchy rash. But that's more or less where the similarities end. Fleas are animals. Ringworm is caused by a fungus. Besides DNA and protein, the two are entirely different. Similarly, bacteria and viruses both have DNA and protein, but have virtually nothing else in common.

Now imagine that every time we treated ringworm with flea medication, the fleas became stronger and did not respond to flea medicine. Soon, we'd have 'super' fleas jumping around, sucking the blood out of people. And all we could do would be to scratch our lesions and hope we don't become anemic. (Not to mention the uproar it would cause with the leech union. Business is bad enough as it is.)

During cold and flu season, the vast majority of coughs, colds, congestions, stuffy noses, runny noses, sore throats and headaches are caused by viral infections. Antibiotics, unfortunately, won't help these illnesses go away. Antibiotics can be helpful if someone has a bacterial infection like strep throat, ear infections, sinusitis, or pneumonia. So how can one tell the difference between a bacterial and a viral infection? That's where your local healthcare providers can help. By asking questions about your symptoms and examining you, they can determine (most of the time) if an infection is caused by a bacteria or a virus.

Unfortunately, some physicians feel pressured to give an antibiotic when they feel it might not be entirely warranted. They perceive, whether real or imagined, that the patient is expecting a prescription for antibiotics. Consider clearing the air ahead of time with your provider by informing him/her that you don't necessarily expect antibiotics, if it's not appropriate.

So by cooperating, communicating openly, and using antibiotics appropriately we can be our own superheroes in the fight against the super bugs. Spandex and masks are optional. This message will self-destruct in five minutes.

Take this Fibro out of My Algia

May 12 was Fibromyalgia Awareness Day. To commemorate the occasion, we should have all pulled an all-nighter helping a friend with large furniture move without the use of any assistive devices. In fact, to make the experience complete, we should have done it with large men who smell like cabbage and chew tobacco. That all-over achy, sleep-deprived feeling we'd all have the next day is how patients with fibromyalgia feel on a good day.

Fibromyalgia (FM) spent many a lonely year on the fringes of medicine. Year after year, it applied for membership in mainstream medical practice and year after year it got rejected for some reason or other (priority being given to more life-threatening diseases, freeze on new enrollment due to budget cuts, invalid username and/or password, etc.) But it was encouraged to apply again in the future. Part of the skepticism by providers regarding FM has been that we don't know what causes it; there are no tests to diagnose it or to determine its severity or progression; and we don't have very effective treatments for it.

The diagnosis is made purely by talking to patients, examining them, and eliminating other possible causes (like being a contestant on Ultimate Fighting Champion).

But recently, more and more, FM has been accepted and recognized as a true ailment. There are still some providers who don't believe it's a true diagnosis, but those numbers are dwindling like bags of rice in a grocery store. (Actually, Costco still has lots of rice in very large bags. They limit it to one or two per customer, but that can be easily circumvented by taking up someone on their 'will work for food' offer, or by making multiple trips to the car with carefully timed application of Groucho Marx glasses—not that I've tried either. And you didn't hear that from me! But I digress.)

The name fibromyalgia is made of 'fibro' meaning having to do with muscle (not dietary) fibers, 'my-' which comes from the root 'myo' meaning muscle, and 'algia' which means pain. In other words, 'fibromyalgia' literally means muscle pain. But it refers to a very specific type of muscle pain. We have all woken up with 'crooks' in our neck from not sleeping right. Imagine having these crooks scattered all over the body every single day. These painful spots—like crooks in the neck—are exquisitely tender.

Patients with FM also don't sleep well which causes constant fatigue. As mentioned before, we don't have very good treatments for it. There are medications that can help, but generally they can only reduce the pain and fatigue, but not eliminate it. It can be a frustrating experience for patients and providers alike.

Even though the cause of FM is unknown, that doesn't mean that we haven't come up with some theories. Some believe it has to do with the sleep disturbance. Others feel that it's brought about by stress. Some believe it's caused by the Loch Ness Monster. Nessie, as insecure as he is, has actually started to wonder if he could be responsible. So much so, that he has started his own 'Cure FM' radio broadcast to raise funds for the National Fibromyalgia Association. (Ironically, the show is broadcast in AM and only in the a.m.)

So FM remains a frontier in medicine. New research is ongoing and hopefully it will bring us newer and better treatments. In the meantime, since we missed the actual FM Awareness Day, perhaps we can spend a month or so being more aware of this disease. After all, I'm sure that's how long a day seems to someone suffering from FM.

A Tale of Two Lovers

'Spring is when a young man's fancy turns to love.' I'm pretty sure I've heard that somewhere, except I'm not sure that sentiment is exclusive to spring. Nonetheless, it serves as a nice segue into this chapter's topic. By segue I mean a smooth transition and not the revolutionary gyroscope-propelled personal transportation device. That is called a Segway. And now we have lost our segue because of the Segway. Perhaps we can hop on our Segway and go look for it!

But I digress.

So a young man's fancy turns to love not just in spring, but pretty much on any day that ends in a 'y'. There are many ways to express love: verbal, emotional, psychological, spiritual, and the much-censored physical.

What makes physical love stand out from all the other forms is its condemnation by the major world religions and its ability to spread disease. (I suppose there are those who would argue that mental illness can be sexually transmitted as well but for now let's pretend it's not.)

Two of the most common types of Sexually Transmitted Diseases (STDs) are gonorrhea and chlamydia.

Gonorrhea and chlamydia have been going out for as long as I can remember. Where one is, it is generally assumed that the other is present, too. They have been together for so long that medical providers refer to them as one entity, GC chlamydia. (The 'GC' stands for GonoCoccus, the official medical name for gonorrhea). Rumor has it that Herpes introduced them!

But as intimate as they are, gonorrhea and chlamydia are not the most flamboyant of diseases. Sure, gonorrhea can give men a thick, disparaging discharge, but for the most part, these two tend to keep a low profile.

A lot of people who have gonorrhea and chlamydia are unaware that they have the infection. Symptoms, when present, can be rather vague: some people have difficulty urinating, some women get a vaginal discharge or pain with intercourse.

That is not to say that gonorrhea and chlamydia are doing charity work in our privates. Far from it! Gonorrhea and chlamydia can cause serious infections in men and women and can render women infertile.

The trouble is that since most people with the disease don't have a lot of symptoms, they can keep spreading the disease without knowing it.

In the past, a swab was needed to check for gonorrhea and chlamydia which discouraged many a man from seeking the diagnosis. But now there is a much less squeam-inducing urine test available.

If someone tests positive for gonorrhea or chlamydia, he/she is given treatment for both, and the partner is treated for both regardless of his/her test results. The couple is also instructed to abstain from physical love until their treatment is complete. Fortunately, the treatment is very short (usually one single dose of an antibiotic or, at most, a week's worth) so the couple can be back frolicking in no time.

In fact, gonorrhea and chlamydia are so common and so difficult to diagnose that most providers are routinely screening all women between the ages of 15 to 24 who are sexually active.

So to all the lovers out there, young and not-as-young, may your lives be filled with love in all its amazing forms. But, if there have been many people whom you've loved, or if you have any symptoms at all, consider getting screened for STDs—especially those two lovers who love 'love', gonorrhea and chlamydia.

Now if I could only find a segue back to the Segway bit . . . .

Thank You, Dr. P

Every time a man complains about how uncomfortable a prostate check is, there is a woman staring at him in disbelief thinking, 'Does your prostate check involve a speculum and a tiny spatula?' Many women undergo the yearly ritual of the Pap smear and it is about as welcome as getting nose hairs plucked by a man with fat fingers.

Some women are quite vocal about their displeasure. One of my medical school classmates once had a female patient look at him accusingly before a pelvic exam and say (referring to the speculum), 'A *man* invented this!' (Apparently, she squinted her eyes and sneered when she said 'maaaaaannn'.) My friend promptly replied, 'I'm not that man.' That day he learned the hard way to agree with anything a woman says during a pelvic exam.

We can all be thankful to a certain man, Dr. Papanicolau. He came up with the idea of scraping some cells from the cervix (the gateway to the uterus—so to speak) by rubbing a small spatula on it and looking at those cells under a microscope to check for cancer. The result was earlier diagnosis and treatment of cervical cancer. The procedure eventually came to bear his name in the truncated form of 'Pap smear'. I don't know if Dr. Papanicolau has any descendents that bear his name, but if he does, my heartfelt sympathy to all the junior high and high school kids in that family. (And you thought *you* got teased because of *your* name!)

Cancer of the cervix used to be one of the leading causes of mortality amongst women. When the Pap smear came along, the number of women who died of cervical cancer dropped dramatically. Nowadays, relatively few women die of it.

Our knowledge of cervical cancer continues to grow. We now know that it is actually a type of Sexually Transmitted Disease (STD). Women who have sex with men are at a much higher risk of getting cervical cancer. (I suppose that's another bullet under the 'pro' column of the Lesbian Association brochure.)

227

Men transmit a virus called Human Papilloma Virus (HPV) to women through intercourse. This virus can cause cancer in the cervix. The more male partners a woman has had in her lifetime (meaning length of life, not the cable channel), the more likely she is to have acquired this virus. Women who have never had intercourse with a man have an exceedingly low incidence of cervical cancer.

The current recommendation for screening is that a woman have a Pap smear within the first three years of becoming sexually active with men, or the age of twenty-one, whichever comes first (kind of like a new car lease agreement). If a woman is monogamous and has had a few normal Pap smears in a row, she can have it done every two to three years—an option many women are more than willing to accept.

In fact, the link between HPV and cervical cancer is so strong that soon we will have a vaccine to prevent it. Hallelujah! However, it's still not a substitute for the Pap smear.

Some women have protested, 'There must be a better way!' Of course there is. We just haven't come up with it yet because, until recently, mostly men had been doing the research on cervical cancer screening. But as we get more women in the field of research, I'm sure they'll come up with less uncomfortable ways to screen for cervical cancer. I suspect we may someday have a simple blood test that will take the place of the Pap smear.

Until then, women will continue to have the 'one up' when it comes to uncomfortable yearly exams. And who knows, these women researchers might come up with a more effective way to screen for prostate cancer that involves biannual ultrasound-guided biopsies through the urethra. Wouldn't that be a change in ways!

There Ought to be a Law

It's the turn of the century (the 20th century) and the town of Springfield, USA is experiencing a population boom.

People know that the town will be world famous one day thanks to the offspring of a certain Mr. Homer Simpson, Sr., and that the cheap lots of land that are now available will soon be worth their weight in Euros.

As the population grows, traffic safety becomes a *must* to avoid accidental deaths and dismemberments. So the City Council, led by the politically ambitious Mr. Quimby, Sr., decides to put up traffic lights at all major intersections. In order to materialize their plan, they turn to the only maker of light bulbs in town, Mr. Montgomery Burns, Jr., a business-savvy young man in his mid-thirties. But at Mr. Burns' prices, they can only afford half the light bulbs they need.

Cries for charity go unheeded. After all, Mr. Burns has to recover his R&D expenses to continue his electronic innovation. 'Do you want to deprive yourselves of life-saving electronic devices in the future?' Mr. Burns declares in a speech. When asked by the press what his true R&D costs are, Mr. Burns simply replies, 'Release the hounds.'

When the townspeople try to import cheaper light bulbs from Canada, Mr. Burns' influence in the Federal Trade Commission (FTC) stymies their efforts. The FTC stated that they could not be certain what the Canadian light bulbs are made of.

Then a certain Mr. Barney Gumble, Sr. comes to town. He, too, can make light bulbs. Mr. Burns, seeing this threat, decides to strike pre-emptively. He gives Mr. Gumble, Sr. a large sum of money to hold off on making light bulbs. Mr. Gumble, Sr. is happy to oblige.

And so, intersections were left unprotected and accidents continued to occur on a regular basis (which was good business for another young entrepreneur, Dr. Nick Rivera, Sr. Although not a medical doctor, Dr. Rivera put his Ph.D. in botany to good use in treating humans. He believed there were few things that a good fertilizer and a stick tied to the trunk wouldn't cure. But I digress.)

While Mr. Burns, Jr.'s act may not be strictly illegal, I feel many would argue that it is ethically shady at best.

We, the people of these United States of America, Jr., are facing a similar situation. There is a bill being stalled in the Senate that would stop 'reverse payments'. A 'reverse payment' is the pharmaceutical equivalent of Mr. Burns, Jr.'s proposition. A brand-name company whose patent is running out pays a generic manufacturer to hold off on making a generic version of their drug, thus enabling the pharmaceutical company to continue to make a profit off the medication.

Naturally, there has been heavy lobbying to oppose this bill that would facilitate the introduction of generic drugs. It's unknown exactly how much money was put forth by the pharmaceutical companies to oppose this bill, but suffice it to say that it would be enough to cover brand-name medications for a small retirement community until the patent runs out.

What's more amazing is that this is not the first time this bill has been stalled. The same thing happened last year.

The senator in question is the brave Senator Kohl of Wisconsin. For some strange reason, he has chosen to forego large campaign contributions and alienate the pharmaceutical industry. I'm sure his story will be told for generations to come: How one man from the Midwest took on Big Pharma and got nowhere with his bill and lost his seat in the Senate and lived the rest of his life regretting his attempt to do the right thing. Big Pharma would then send his picture to all other senators as a subtle reminder of the consequences of trying to take on Big Pharma.

But just as the town of Springfield eventually overcame its traffic light problem, we, the people of these United States of America, Jr., shall overcome our drug problem, too. As far as our real-estate woes are concerned, I'm afraid we're on our own.

(*Editor's Note*: Looks like the second district court ruled that reverse payments are not anti-trust. So sounds like it'll continue. Here's the link in case you're curious.)
http://www.ipwatchdog.com/2010/04/29/reverse-payments-not-antitrust-violation/id=10339/

Think BIG Avocado (Choking)

The Avocado Festival has a long and glorious tradition in the Carpinteria area. It dates back to the Mesozoic era when cavemen gathered all along the main road, selling saber-toothed tiger pelts, reprints of cave drawings, and enjoying some live grunting and rock music (meaning music made by rocks—not rock-and-roll).

But now it's time to branch out. It's time to go national. And what better way to get the nation's attention than a bit of sensational journalism. I'm going to send an article to every single Times/Bugle/Tribune/Daily/Press publication out there with the headline, 'Avocado Lovers Risk Peril at Carpinteria Avocado Festival'. The article, naturally, would be about the risk of choking.

As far as I understand it, when writing a sensationalistic piece, the frequency of an event is not very important. After all, a headline that reads, '300 Million Doses of Medication were Administered Today Without Error', is hardly attention grabbing. So while the risk of choking at an event like the Avocado Festival is quite low, we can still do a piece on it to grab the nation's attention.

Choking is when food goes down the 'wind pipe', commonly known as the 'trachea'. The 'food pipe' and the 'wind pipe' are dangerously close together in the human throat—or the throats of most animals, for that matter. To compensate, there is an elaborate system of pulleys, shutters, valves, and crossing guards that all work together to get the food to the food pipe and away from the wind pipe. (Frankly, I'm surprised we haven't seen more lawsuits against Mother Nature for such a blatantly faulty design. I would have expected a recall or, at the very least, a software upgrade!)

So the swallow mechanism isn't exactly fool proof. Sometimes lines get crossed and things go down the wrong pipe.

When wind goes down the food pipe, it's hardly a grave concern. The air will escape the stomach/intestines one way or another. But when food goes down the wind pipe, that is a much more dire situation. The body does very poorly without oxygen.

A victim is considered to be choking if he/she cannot breathe, speak, or cough. If any of the above are possible, the airway is not completely blocked and, most of the time, the victim can get the food out on their own. Patting the victim on the back can help the bystander feel useful.

If the victim is unable to speak, cough, or breathe, then it's important to intervene.

A very popular and effective method is the Heimlich maneuver. This technique is demonstrated in many movies such as 'Mrs. Doubtfire'. (In the final scene in the restaurant, Robin Williams does it on Pierce Brosnan.) It involves approaching the victim from behind, placing the thumb-side of a fist just above the belly button, placing the other hand on the pinkie side of the fist and giving strong upward thrusts. Any CPR class has a choking section complete with dummies for practice.

People most commonly choke on solid foods. Children can choke on small objects (anything smaller than their fist), such as toys and coins. Hotdogs can also be a choking risk for children under three years of age if they take a bite out of a hotdog. Cutting the hot dog into small pieces before it goes into little mouths can help.

So let's start getting ready for an even bigger Avocado Festival in the years to come! I envision Palestinians and Israelis, French and Brits, and North Koreans and South Koreans all dipping their taquitos in the same guacamole dip. In the meantime, let's all get CPR-certified so that, in case someone chokes, we can intervene. That would lead to even more articles which would lead to even more exposure which would lead to an even bigger Avocado Festival! One world, one Avocado Festival!

Ugly Stomach-Intestin-itis

For those of you playing the 'For the Health of It!' home game, I would argue that this chapter would not qualify as a DAISNAID (Do As I Say, Not As I Do.) Do you remember the chapter called 'Chill Out on Fever'? (Of course you don't; you read so many books, it's hard to keep track.) In that chapter, we talked about how a fever, in and of itself, is not a bad thing and that if the fever-ridden person is not uncomfortable, it is not necessary to treat the fever.

My almost one-year-old son came down with a fever recently, and we did treat his fever. But in all fairness, he was pretty uncomfortable. And when baby's uncomfortable, mommy and daddy are uncomfortable. And when mommy and daddy are uncomfortable, the cat's uncomfortable because we're not fully at her beck and call. And when the cat's uncomfortable, the furniture gets scratched. So for our furniture, and the baby's comfort, we treated his fever.

He also had foul-smelling diarrhea. (Normally, his diarrhea smells like rosemary and cumin.) He was suffering from acute viral gastroenteritis. Don't let the name fool you, there's nothing cute about it—even when it affects really cute babies. 'Gastro' refers to the stomach. 'Entero' means intestines. And 'itis' means inflammation. Put them together and that spells stomach and intestine inflammation.

This type of infection is commonly known as the 'stomach flu'. It is not to be confused with the respiratory flu for which we have a vaccine. So if a person who received the flu vaccine gets the 'stomach flu', it's not a sign of the vaccine's failure. It's just a sign of the medical community's vocabulary conflicting with the non-medical community's vocabulary. Although, that is of little consolation when one is in the throes of gastric upheaval.

The intestinal flu virus enters the body through the mouth via contaminated food, hands, drink, hands, objects, hands, and objects. Once in the stomach, the virus starts to cause inflammation. An inflamed stomach causes nausea, vomiting and fever. Then the battle starts. The immune system rushes in to fight off the virus and the chase is on. After a day or two, the virus is chased out of the stomach and the nausea and diarrhea resolve.

The virus then runs to the intestines (no pun intended) with the immune cells in hot, smelly pursuit. The intestines become inflamed and start to spasm and cause diarrhea. Due to the immense length of the intestines, this chase can take three to five days.

Once the virus hits the end of the intestines, the immune system kicks it out and the illness is gone. The good news is that the immune system is fully capable of dealing with this illness. The bad news is that it takes about a week for all of it to happen and we have no medications to help it along.

Our duty as vessels of the intestines is to make sure we stay well-hydrated by drinking lots of fluids. A good way to tell the vessel's hydration status is how often one needs to empty the urinary cargo holds. If it's four times a day, hydration status is good. Full steam ahead! Scrub the decks! Deck the halls! (But not before Thanksgiving.)

Once the stomach feels better, it starts to ask for food. In spite of what the stomach requests, one should realize that the stomach is still not fully recovered. One should start with the BRAT diet (Bananas, Rice, Applesauce and Toast), since these foods are easier to digest, and gradually add regular foods. It would be wise to add meat and dairy last since they're harder to digest.

So here's hoping none of us gets first-hand/gastroenteric experience with the stomach flu. (Hand-washing is the most effective way to do so.) If we do, fluids, rest, and the BRAT diet can help get us through. However, if we are not urinating at least four times a day, or if the diarrhea is bloody, then it warrants further evaluation because it has gone beyond the realm of routine gastroenteritis. In that case, see your healthcare provider for further instructions.

Up All Night Asleep

On December 21st, the winter solstice is upon us. Winter solstice, being the longest night of the year, is a joyous occasion for night owls. Come to think of it, it's also a joyous occasion for day owls since it means the days will be getting longer. So there should be joy all around.

Before the invention of fire by Fire and Associates, Inc., I imagine early humans must have slept a lot on this night. Afterall, I doubt their television programming would have been much to stay up for.

These days, we have the luxury of choosing how much of this longest night we spend asleep, unless one suffers from Obstructive Sleep Apnea (OSA).

To understand sleep apnea, we must first understand the sleep cycle. There are four stages of sleep, aptly named stages one through four. I like to think of them as sleep gears. Sleep gears one and two are light sleep. These are the gears that get the sleep started from the dead-stop of wakefulness.

Sleep gears three and four are the deep restful stages. They are the cruising gears of sleep. These gears move us through the deep sleep that make us feel rested and refreshed. (These are also the gears that brighten eyes and bushify tails, if one is so inclinced.)

During sleep stages three and four, all the muscles in the body, including the ones in the throat, relax. In some people, this relaxation causes the back part of the roof of the mouth to collapse onto the tongue, blocking the airway. The sound of air passing through this collapsed passage is known as snoring. But in some people, the collapse is so strong that air cannot pass at all. These people actually stop breathing for a few seconds during deep sleep. This stoppage in breathing is called sleep apnea. It is also a very common cause of panic in bedfellows as they wait seemingly endless seconds to see if breathing will resume.

Due to pre-arranged contractual agreements between body functions, breathing gets priority over all others. If our body functions were patrons

235

waiting outside a dance club on a cold winter solstice night, sleep would be the guy who gets dropped off by his driver, walks right up to the front of the line, and is promptly and courteously let in by the muscular bouncer with the surprisingly soft hands. (What does he put on them?)

When the brain senses that air is not moving, it downshifts the body out of deep sleep and into light sleep, thereby robbing the sleep apnea sufferer of the restful stages of sleep.

An hour or so later, the brain tries to go into deep sleep again and the cycle repeats itself throughout the night. Meanwhile, the sleep apnea sufferer is completely unaware of this cycling in and out of deep sleep. As far as they're concerned, they've slept through the night. And yet, they still feel sleepy the next day.

The fact that breathing gets top billing amongst bodily functions does not mean that sleep waits idly by. Since the body is sleep deprived, it tries to get sleep when it can. People with sleep apnea find that they fall asleep during quiet activities, such as reading or watching television. They also nod off very quickly when they're a passenger in a car.

So when we commemorate this longest night of the year, may we all enjoy the deep restful sleep we deserve so we may be rested and alert to face the ever-lengthening days. But if our loved ones (or neighbors down the street) complain about our snoring and wait in terror through our apneic spells, a visit to our primary care provider may be in order. He/she can help us decipher if our symptoms are from sleep apnea. If they are, treatments are available. But that's a topic for a future chapter—maybe the summer solstice one.

Vertigo

'And thus Frodo wandered, through the Pinna, into the External Auditory Meatus. He pierced through the membranous wall of the Tympanum and scaled the Incus, Stapes, and Malleus until he reached the Utricle. There, casting a shadow up on the Cochlea, stood the three semi-circular canals that rule proprioception. They were arranged just as the legend had described, facing all possible directions: north to south, east to west and up and down.

'The semi-circular canals had been angered. They had brought vertigo upon the land. They had caused movement without movement, bringing new chapters to the Chronicles of Nauseum. And now the body faced the possible awakening of the dreaded Vomitus.'

That's the opening of my planned fourth volume to the Lord of the Rings Trilogy. After all, any good consumer will tell you that if 'one ring to rule them all' is good, then three rings must be ten times better. And if there can be a sequel to *Friday the 13th: the Final Chapter*, then so can there be a fourth part to a trilogy. But I digress.

The three semi-circular canals of the inner ear are, indeed, the rulers of proprioception. 'Proprioception' is the body's ability to tell it is moving even when the eyes are closed. Try it in action: Sit in a swivel chair. Close your eyes. Ask someone to rotate the chair. You will be able to tell which way the chair is turning. That's proprioception. (On the other hand, if someone important is coming to town and they are greeted and treated appropriately, that is called a 'proper reception'. People experience propriception during a proper reception, but not necessarily vice versa.) Now, where was I?

So the semi-circular canals tell us when our bodies are moving. This is part of the reason why people get motion sickness (see chapter herein). What enables them to do that is fluid. Each semi-circular canal—as most canals are—is filled with fluid. As the head moves, the fluid shifts within the canal, gently caressing tiny microscopic hairs inside which then send a signal of movement to the brain. This is very similar to how ocean currents move amber fields of kelp.

Sometimes, for various reasons, the canals get inflamed. When they get inflamed, they start to malfunction, sending signals of movement to the brain even when the body is still. This is called vertigo—the feeling that the body is in motion when it is not. People experience this as a spinning sensation that comes on with changes in head position, such as turning over in bed or sitting up from a lying position.

Some people have microscopic crystals floating in the fluid of their semi-circular canals. These crystals can settle on the microscopic hairs in the canal, much like trash from a cruise ship gliding down onto those amber fields of kelp. When these crystals make contact with the microscopic hairs, a signal of movement is sent to the brain. The brain feels obliged to acknowledge the signal and makes the body feel like it's moving.

There is a medication called meclizine that can help slow down the spinning part of vertigo. It's available over the counter. The drawback is that it makes people very sleepy and thus doesn't exactly increase one's functionality.

There are exercises that can reposition the crystal and 'reset' the system. These can be helpful in people who have the microscopic crystals in their inner ear. Your local healthcare provider can help.

So will Frodo tame the inflamed semi-circular canals by retrieving the crystals? Will that bring peace back to the land? Will he ever find shoes with a wide enough toe box to match his smock? You'll just have to wait for the book-signing tour. I must go now. I'm expecting a call from Peter Jackson.

Viva Avocado!

Look! Up on that tree!
It's a black pear!
It's a large fig!
No! It's an avocado!!

Faster than a speeding bullet (when shot out of a cannon at speeds faster than a speeding bullet)! More powerful than a locomotive (if you put a bunch of their seeds on the tracks)! Able to leap tall buildings in a single shot out of a cannon (see above)! Champion of justice and the American Way (and by American I mean Aztec not Anglo-Saxon)!

Yes, it's Avocado Festival time in Carpinteria. Sure, Goleta has its lemon festival, and Santa Barbara may boast its French, Greek, Italian, and Sri-Lankan festivals, but the Avocado Festival in Carpinteria is the greatest large-single-hard-seed-fruit-related festival this side of Sheffield Exit, north of Seacliff Drive, west of the ocean and east of the Santa Ynez mountains.

Around this time of year, the main drag gets filled with any and all methods to enjoy the avocado: Take a dip in the World's Largest Vat of Guac. (I mean using a chip, not the body. I'm sure diving into the World's Largest Vat of Guac is highly illegal, regardless of how fun it is.)

Stop by for a scoop of avocado ice cream. Try on some avocado clothing. Take a pet avocado home—it's wonderful with kids. (Just don't let the dog near it.)

I'd like to think that the avocado got its name from the Spanish word for lawyer, 'abogado', because the Native Americans found it to be a particularly just fruit. (I'd also like to think that I could bend a spoon with my mind force, but that doesn't necessarily make it so.)

The avocado does, however, get its name from the way it hangs in pairs off the tree. Apparently, when the Native American men saw it on the tree, it reminded them of a certain body part of theirs and thus they believed it to be endowed with aphrodisiac properties.

Whilst the aphrodisiac properties of the avocado have not proven to be true, it does have other health benefits.

Avocados can lower LDL, aka bad cholesterol, while maintaining HDL, aka good cholesterol. (For more information on cholesterol, see chapter herein.) It does this through the power of 'plant sterols'. Some astute readers might notice that 'cholesterol' contains the word 'sterol'. As it turns out, the 'chole' part is exclusive to animals; therefore, plants do not have cholesterol. But they do have their own version, collectively known as 'plant sterols'.

'Plant sterols' can lower cholesterol. The spreads in the grocery store that are emblazoned with the red, starburst label that says 'Helps reduce cholesterol' can claim that because they are made with plant sterols. And our friend, the avocado, has it.

Avocados are also rich in fiber, folate, vitamins C and E, and potassium. That's virtually a multivitamin in itself! (I'd like to see Centrum Silver pull *that* off and still be so tasty on a turkey sandwich!)

The orange fanatics and banana lovers might respectively claim that their respective fruits have vitamin C and potassium, respectively. But with all due respect, did either of those fruits inspire Native American men to love?

Enjoying avocados in moderation would be best (i.e., best not to dive into the World's Largest Vat of Guac) since they have about 300 calories each. That's the equivalent of two shot glasses of olive oil.

And now it's time to put on our sombreros and sing along (to the tune of 'Canta No Llores'). Ay yay yay yay, viva Avocado. Que buen es el gusto y rico sabor. No quiero menudo donde es amor? But I digress.

Special thanks to Chantal Gariepy, Registered Dietician with Sansum Clinic, for providing the facts about avocados.

Watch the Sleds!

Thank goodness the holiday season arrives every year! How else would we endure the long, harsh, cold, bitter California winter when the highs dip as low as 60? This time of festivity always comes just in time to lift our weary spirits as we prepare for our annual holiday barbecue.

Auld acquaintances are forgot and never brought to mind. (I think that's ancient Celtic for 'We have to invite Uncle John to the party because he invited us to his son's bar mitzvah.') Homes and work places are filled with decorative items and lots and lots and lots of sweets and treats.

Some find this quite distressing. The devil on the left shoulder urges them to indulge and binge on things from which they are trying to abstain. The angel on the right shoulder is suspiciously silent. Is she wiping cookie crumbs off of her face? Oh, come on!

People's approaches to the holiday eating dilemma are as diverse as recipes for fruit cake. Some don't even bother to try. They concede defeat right before Thanksgiving, allowing themselves to be washed away in a wave of gourmandize. They simply try to keep their head above water until the New Year dietary reset button starts in six weeks. Others try to build up 'food credit' by skipping meals leading up to a big event.

The end result tends to be gained weight during the holidays which people try to lose after the New Year—with mixed success.

Unfortunately, there is no magical cure for this holiday gustatory and gastronomic quandary. (The previous phrasing brought to you by my word-of-the-day calendar. I'm in the 'G' section.) But all is not lost! It is possible to approach the holidays with a somewhat more proactive attitude.

Let's imagine that the body is Santa's workshop and calories are toys. If there are more toys coming into the workshop than toys being given out, the workshop will need to make more room and thus become larger.

But toys come in different sizes. It takes a lot more yo-yos (meaning the toy with the string that goes up and down, not someone who lacks street smarts) to fill the workshop than it does sleds. (Sleds are wooden transportation devices used in snowy areas. Apparently, they slip on snow and people can use them to get down inclines. See any winter depiction by Norman Rockwell for a visual.)

In the food world, this is known as 'calorie density'. A piece of lettuce would be considered a yo-yo because it doesn't have a lot of calories, i.e., only one calorie. One slice of pecan pie would be considered a sled because it has 500 calories.

So if Santa wanted to keep his workshop the same size through the tempting holiday season, he would be wise to watch how many sleds he lets in. Not to say that Santa can't have any sleds (especially the kinds with ice cream on top)—it's just that he might want to have fewer of them.

Let's look at it from a numbers perspective: A pound of fat contains 3500 calories. It would take 3500 leaves of lettuce to gain a pound; whereas it would take only seven slices of pecan pie to accomplish the same gain.

So every meal and snack time could be an opportunity. If the item is calorie dense, i.e., cookies, candies, pie, etc., consider limiting the portion. If the item is less calorie dense, i.e., salad, vegetables, consider having more of it.

Also, consider having the less calorie-dense items first. They take up space in the workshop and thus can help in portion control with the calorie-rich items.

So here's wishing everyone a happy holiday season! Good luck! And I'll see you at the gym on January 2.

Water Safety

Summertime is here! How do I know? I saw it on 'The Daily Show'. It's my number one source for news, weather, stocks and health. On the show, it said that the days are longer, the weather is warmer, kids are out of school, and thus people all over the country have started engaging in leisurely activities, many of which involve water.

Exposure to water, as enjoyable as it is, can be hazardous. One of those hazards, Swimmer's Ear, was discussed in 'The Aural Trilogy' chapter herein. There are, however, other more serious hazards of water exposure.

I fretted long and hard about doing a chapter on water safety, specifically because it would involve discussing drowning. It's such a morose subject, yet it is so important—especially since a bit of preparation and awareness can greatly reduce the risk. So I decided to not use the word 'drowning' at all. For the purposes of this topic, I shall give it another name: 'Steve'. So whenever you see the word 'Steve' in this article, know that it refers to (whisper) 'drowning'.

Our history with water goes way back to our primitive single-celled predecessors who lived in primordial earth. Talk about a simpler time! Food was absorbed directly through the skin (although back then we would have called it the 'cell membrane', except that we didn't have vocal cords). We reproduced by splitting ourselves in two, which involved virtually no pain or midwives. Since we were all single-celled organisms, there was no 'Stem Cell' controversy. And there were no 'other genders' to contend with. Back then, water was our medium of choice. We lived, ate, slept, pooped and reproduced in it.

Admittedly, there are people who still eat, sleep, poop, and reproduce in water but to a much lesser extent than our primordial distant, *distant* cousins.

Water is still a very large part of our lives, but our contact with it is more intermittent. Being vigilant during those intermittent contacts can make for a much safer experience with 'the liquid of life'.

The first step is prevention. This means blocking unintended access to bodies of water. Fences around pools with a gate that closes and latches automatically work best. (Be sure the latch is taller than any small children, or put a lock on it.) It is important to monitor children closely at beaches, lakes, and wading pools. In fact, even a bucket of water used for mopping can be a danger if a toddler happens to stumble upon it and get his/her head stuck in it. A toilet bowl can cause the same hazard. So keeping the house clear of water containers and blocking unwanted access to bathrooms and toilet bowls can help.

Step two is knowing what to do if Steve occurs. Fortunately, the hair on our bodies and the two little targets on our chests place us in the great class of 'mammals'. One of the perks of being a mammal is that we are endowed with the 'mammalian diving reflex'. When a mammal is submerged in water for too long, its body goes into a protective mode. Blood is moved away from the extremities and towards the 'vital organs', such as the brain, heart, lungs, and intestines. This effectively helps to sustain life for a longer period. The colder the water is, the stronger the reflex.

This is where knowing CPR can be very helpful. When someone's been under water too long, especially in cold water, performing CPR and warming the body can help revive the victim. The American Red Cross has many classes for infant, child, and adult CPR. They run throughout the summer. Their website, *www.redcross.org*, has more information on times and locations.

So here's wishing everyone a happy and safe summer. Let's enjoy our return to the liquid that first made life possible. By being prepared and aware, may we have nothing but fond memories of water sports, sunshine, sweet cool treats (in moderation, of course), and spending time with family and friends. And to all the 'Steves' out there (the real Steves, not the euphemisms for drowning), I apologize if this article has caused any confusion.

Weight Loss Correlations

During the last whirlwind presidential campaign, there was a lot of talk about Main Street. (The only Main Street I know is the one at Disneyland, but I don't think that's what the candidates were referring to because there was no mention of a magic shop or a movie theater that plays Steamboat Willie endlessly.)

I've come to suspect that Main Street is a way for politicians to refer to 'regular Americans'. And I'm almost certain that 'regular', in this context, does not refer to bowel habits. Perhaps 'regular' refers to the most common type of people—like those with internal skeletons and warm blood.

Sitting in my home on Secondary Drive, I imagine that a lot of people on Main Street are looking to become healthier by eating better and exercising more in the coming year.

So in order to help my brethren on Main Street, I've compiled a list of characteristics that are correlated with achieving and maintaining a healthy weight. Some keen readers might point out that correlation does not imply causation (see chapter herein). To them I say, 'Touché, my good man (or woman)! How about some brandy?'

While it is true that just because a behavior is correlated with weight loss, it doesn't mean that it *causes* weight loss, the behaviors we will review here certainly do not cause any harm and can be beneficial for overall health and well-being regardless of their effect on weight.

So here they are, in no particular order:

Sleep: People who get adequate sleep (seven to eight hours a night) tend to maintain healthier weights. This may seem counterintuitive since if one is awake, one is clearly more active than when one is sleeping and thus must burn more calories. The counter to this counter-intuition is that people universally eat more when awake than when sleeping (except certain people on zolpidem [Ambien]). Also, sleep is a very complex process that involves many hormonal controls that seem to have an effect on weight.

Getting adequate sleep also helps people stay mentally sharp and makes learning easier. So even if one does not lose weight, at least one will be more mentally clear about their weight problem.

Eating slowly: People who eat slowly also tend to maintain healthy weights. They also have fewer problems with acid reflux (heartburn). In order to facilitate this behavior, consider playing the 'Hands Down, Fork Down' game. Here are the rules: All people at the table must put their hands and/or fork down while chewing and must wait until they've swallowed before taking another bite. If one is caught stuffing their mouth before it's empty, the spotter gets a point. At the end of the meal, whoever has accrued the most points wins! (Beware of using desserts as prizes.) If someone makes a comment about how slow one is eating, it is important to work the word 'masticate' into the response.

If one is eating alone, one can still play the game and keep a personal record of the number of bites taken before the previous one has been swallowed. (In this case, one would try to get the lowest score possible.)

Using smaller dishes: There was a study done with dieticians where one group used regular dishes, the other group used smaller dishes, and the caloric intake of each group was monitored. It was noted that the dieticians who used smaller dishes consumed less calories. If a dietician, who is an expert on proportions and calories, is affected by dish size, what chance do the rest of us mortals have? (Another benefit of using smaller dishes is that one can buy them real cheap at IKEA. They come in a variety of colors and are made of plastic and are thus unbreakable when one smashes them on the ground in celebration of becoming the 'Hands Down, Fork Down' champion! But I digress.)

So here's wishing everyone on Main Street, Secondary Drive, and Insignificant Cul-de-sac a happy and healthy life. May our rejuvenant, vibrant bodies become a model for our economy. And may we do it without a bailout.

Well-Defined Lungs and Nostrils

When the average person thinks of steroids, they envision an overly muscular man or woman who has become an evolutionary dead end. Others picture people with puffy cheeks, round bellies, and sky-high blood sugars who are walking time-bombs of heart disease. Steroids are indeed powerful things. They can cause great benefits and great harm. Most people have a healthy fear and apprehension when it comes to using steroids.

These days, at least in certain cases, we have been able to harness the healing power of steroids and avoid all the nasty side effects. By 'we' I mean the R&D team of your favorite drug manufacturer. They have breathed new life into the treatment of asthma and allergies. (Pun intended)

When I was a student at UC Santa Barbara, I remember carrying a tissue around with me all the time. My eyes were puffy and blood shot. I looked tired and I was constantly blowing my nose. Everyone who saw me thought I had been crying. They would try to console me by saying that they, too, had a hard time in Art History 6A. 'All of those Medieval Churches look alike!' they would say. In reality, failing the test was the least of my worries. I couldn't breathe!

As if that wasn't enough, one day after exercising, I got a wheeze that didn't go away for days. I walked over to student health and was informed that I have asthma. I almost thought the doctor was making it up. I'd never had asthma before. I'd seen asthmatics in movies. They were gaunt, pale, and hunched over all the time gasping for breath. That wasn't me.

I struggled with various treatment regimens, most of which I never used consistently. My mother was on a nasal steroid which she lent to me, but I just didn't get it. It didn't make sense to me to use something that didn't work right away. I had to use it for four or five days for it to work. What a lazy medicine!

Medical school brought temporary relief. Apparently, Milwaukee has an entirely different flora than Santa Barbara. My naïve immune system wasn't used to Milwaukee pollen and so it didn't react to it. But I soon realized that medical school in the Midwest is a rather expensive treatment for asthma and allergies. There had to be a better way.

It wasn't until after residency that I really started taking my asthma and allergies seriously. I'm proud to say that now, I sniff and inhale steroids daily. (Yes! It's true!) My lungs and nostrils have never felt better. I'm still not terribly muscular. I don't have puffy cheeks or a round belly. Yet I still reap all the benefits of being on a steroid.

So my message to all the asthma and allergy sufferers is this: embrace the steroid if it comes in a spray. Be assured that you have at your disposal the healing power of the good genie of the steroid lamp. Be further assured that the evil genie cannot access your body through your nose or lungs. We shall suffer no more!

Which Doctor Would You Ask to Pick Out a Watermelon?

Everyone knows it's important to look good while picking out a watermelon. Here's the sequence as recommended by WAAK (Watermelon Acquirer Association, oK?): Pick up a watermelon, smell it, hold it to your ear, pretend to be shocked and quickly put it back in the bin burying it near the bottom. Pick another watermelon, hold the melon firmly in one hand and pat with the pads of the fingers of the other hand, put it in your shopping cart, whisper something to it, pretend to walk away and then quickly double back (repeat as necessary).

Of that entire sequence, patting the watermelon is what really helps to determine a good watermelon. The act of tapping the watermelon and interpreting it is called 'percussion'. It's the same word that's used for the section of a band where the guy that's a little 'off' pounds away on various hollow objects and then proceeds to eat the drum sticks at the end of the show.

Doctors use percussion when examining patients. We've all the seen the classic sequence (either in person or in the media): the doctor places the middle finger of one hand on the patient's abdomen or chest, and taps it with the tip of the middle finger of the other hand.

Much like the watermelon case, 'percussing' gives important information. Mainly, it tells if things are solid or hollow. For example, normally, the lungs are filled with air and thus should sound hollow. But if there is water around the lungs, they will sound solid when percussed.

The same can be said about the liver which usually hides underneath the ribs on the right side of the abdomen. Tapping on the soft part of the abdomen on the right side should sound hollow because of the intestines. But if the liver is enlarged and sticking out from under the ribs, the area will sound solid.

Doctors who deal with things inside the chest or abdomen (like primary care physicians, pulmonologists and gastroenterologists) use percussion more regularly. Other specialists, like ophthalmologists or radiologists, do not since

250 Ali Javanbakht, M.D.

X-rays look the same whether or not they're percussed, and percussing the eye can actually make the situation worse.

Besides the mere presence of fluid around the lungs or an enlarged liver, percussion can help determine how *much* fluid is around the lungs and how much a liver is enlarged. A doctor can use percussion to determine where the solid sound becomes hollow and thus locate the edge of the liver or level of fluid in the lungs.

As helpful as percussion can be in making a diagnosis, it's still not as precise as an X-ray of the lungs or an ultrasound of the abdomen in determining the extent of a disease. So a confirmatory test is usually done to follow up on abnormal percussion.

So the next time one is in the grocery store looking for a good watermelon, one can try grabbing the abdomen, collapsing to the floor and yelling, 'Ow, my liver! I think it's enlarging again! Can anyone percuss it?' (At which point, the store's PA system would bellow, 'Is there a doctor in the house?') Once the health provider has demonstrated good percussing technique, one can casually turn the conversation towards watermelons: 'All this excitement has made me thirsty. A good, ripe watermelon sure sounds good right now. Which one do you recommend?'

This may sound like a lot to go through to get a good watermelon, but to me, it's well worth it. There's nothing worse than coming home and opening a perfectly good-looking watermelon only to find it slimy and over-ripe or pale and under-ripe inside. Life's too short and the summer's even shorter.

Worth a Shot

As the long days of summer wind down, and the old watering hole dries up (because we never got around to getting that crack in the swimming pool fixed), families across the country start the sacred ritual of going 'Back to School'.

In fact, from what I remember as a teenager, it seemed like 'Back to School' started the week after school was out! That's about when I'd start seeing mailers about the Back-to-School Sale at K-Mart. I found it rather infuriating, but then again, in those turbulent teenage years, it didn't take much. I remember having an internal tantrum when *Moonlighting* was cancelled. What made it worse was that I never gathered the courage to admit to any of my friends—who all watched *Miami Vice*—that I was a *Moonlighting* fan. Thus, I mourned in silence.

Besides precocious department store sales and cancelled TV shows, some families' back-to-school repertoires involve some kind of contact with their healthcare provider. This is most evident with the kindergartners who need to have a physical and a form filled out before starting school. And every kindergartner's most favoritest thing about getting a physical—besides the poking, prodding, and inspection of privates—is the shots. And we in the healthcare industry certainly haven't helped matters much by scheduling them for no fewer than five needle pokes: three vaccinations, one anemia check and a skin test for tuberculosis.

The typical kindergartner gets a vaccine for diphtheria, tetanus, and whooping cough (combined in one shot), measles, mumps and rubella (combined in one shot), and polio. Since polio doesn't play well with other vaccines, it has to sit in a syringe all by itself and think about what it's done. It may come back when it's ready to play nice with the other vaccines.

After kindergarten, there's a lull in vaccinations until the twelve-year visit. At that time, children are due for a tetanus booster. But the wonderful vaccine manufacturers of America have developed a whooping cough booster that is scheduled for the twelve-year visit as well! 'But freteth not ye pre-teens', as the Bard would say (if the term pre-teen had been available during his time), these same vaccine manufacturers had the foresight to combine it with the tetanus vaccine so you still get only one shot. But don't stop fretting entirely! The CDC has just added a new vaccine to the schedule for the twelve-year physical, the meningococcal vaccine. So it will be two shots for the twelve-year-olds after all.

The meningococcal vaccine, as the name suggests, protects against a certain kind of meningitis caused by the *meningococcus* bacteria. This is not to be confused with a *political caucus*, which I believe has to do with real estate. Both can be potentially bad for your health.

Meningitis is an infection of the sack that surrounds the spine and brain. Previously, this vaccine was recommended for college students and people in army barracks because the illness spreads quickly to people in close quarters and it tends to infect younger people. But now, the CDC expanded it to all twelve-year-olds entering junior high—the reason being that meningitis caused by meningococcus progresses very rapidly. A patient can go from the first symptoms of the illness to being critically ill or even dying within 24 to 72 hours. What makes it especially challenging is that, by the time someone is ill enough to seek treatment, it can be too late and antibiotics might not work. The one-time meningococcal vaccine is our best chance against this illness.

So, kindergartners and twelve-year-olds, gather your parents and head towards your primary care provider's office. Ask to be protected against diseases. Show your parents the foresight and perspective you possess deep down inside. They will be very impressed, because I'm sure very few of them (myself included) had that kind of foresight when they were your age. But that was probably because we had to walk to school twelve miles, uphill, backwards, in the snow, both ways, in the middle of July while fighting off a pack of rabid wolves using nothing but loose-leaf notebook paper and a piece of gum. (Be sure they promise to buy you a toy afterwards!)

Your Epidermis is Showing

Showing your epidermis is nothing to be ashamed of. (Or as my high school English teacher would have me say, 'That's nothing of which to be ashamed'). I show my epidermis all the time! I'm showing it right now—as are you, reading this chapter.

Epidermis is the medical term for skin—specifically, the very top layer of skin. There's a wonderful billboard that the Australians have made that features some young, good-looking, muscular, and unnaturally hairless men standing naked with their hands in front of them like groomsmen at a wedding ceremony. The caption reads, 'Protect your largest organ'. It was an ad for promoting the use of sunscreen. The skin is, indeed, the body's largest organ.

With summer now in full swing, there will be many an epidermis getting sun exposure. Most people know that exposure to the sun increases the risk of skin cancer. It also makes the skin darker and more wrinkly.

Most people know it's a good idea to use sunscreen and wide-brimmed hats to protect their skin from the sun. Wearing long-sleeved shirts and pants is helpful, too, but it's hard to find the motivation to dress up that way to go to the beach on a hot day. Most people are also conscientious enough to buy sunscreen with a high enough SPF (15 or higher) and to get the 'all day/water proof/sport/NASA-tested' variety to protect themselves better.

What most people don't know is what the SPF stands for. I was one of those people. I could tell you that it stands for Sniff Pink Furniture, but I'd be lying. (And we all know that it's better to sit than to lie.) So I will sit here and tell you that the SPF tells you how much time the sunscreen gives you before you get burned.

The way SPF is determined is that they take volunteers, have some of them put on a specific sunscreen, expose all of them to the sun or UV radiation and see how much longer it takes the sunscreen people to get burned. So if the non-sunscreen people burn in ten minutes and the sunscreen people burn in fifty minutes, then the SPF is 5.

This process is used to determine SPF up to 15. Since no one wants to sit under a UV light for ten hours, so SPF's higher than 15 aren't actually measured. It's an 'extrapolation'—meaning that the manufacturers assume that doubling the sun-protective ingredient in an SPF 15 sunscreen will increase its SPF to 30.

The important point to bear in mind is that it has never been determined that sunscreens *prevent* sunburns. They simply delay it.

Also, even the waterproof/sweatproof/Sporty Spice sunscreen loses effectiveness with exposure to water and sweat. (It is unclear if exposure to Sporty Spice itself has any effect on the wearer, but it can't possibly be good for anyone's health.) So there are many factors that can reduce protection from sunscreen.

Imagine you're out fishing around the Channel Islands and you hit an iceberg. The hole in the bottom of the boat causing it to sink is like the sun trying to burn your skin. The bait-bucket (now empty because you dumped all the bait overboard to use the bucket to get water out of the boat and, wouldn't you know it—all of a sudden, the fish are just jumping out of the water! It figures!) is like sunscreen. Sweat and water exposure are like the leaks from the rust on the bottom of the bucket (because your 'friend' didn't rinse the seawater out of the bucket the last time he borrowed it). On particularly hot days, that hole in the boat can be quite large and no bucket of any size can prevent the boat from sinking.

So the cornerstone of sun protection is limiting sun exposure. A good rule of thumb is to spend fifteen minutes of every hour in the shade. (A good rule of the big toe is to cut the nail square instead of curved to avoid ingrown toenails. Bonus advice at no extra charge. It's the summer special! But I digress.)

As the saying goes: An ounce of prevention is worth two in the bush. Taking the time to practice good sun protection can yield great rewards later in life, such as reduced need for surgery and less wrinkles, thus resulting in a healthier, happier epidermis.

Your Lungs on 'Roids

If I had been a doctor forty years ago, I'd be really old today. I could reminisce about how back then, medicine was simpler, with hardly any bureaucracy or paperwork. As an example, I would talk about asthma. Back then, when patients with asthma would come to see me, the visit would be rather short. 'Avoid things that trigger your asthma. If you get an attack, shoot yourself with epinephrine. Have a nice day.' I would leave the exam room and have my nurse educate the patient or parent on how to administer epinephrine at home. She would encourage the adult patients to have a list of projects handy for the boost of energy the shots bring and warn children's parents to remove all sharp objects and pad the walls.

Nowadays, the asthma visit is a big production, complete with color-coded inhalers and devices to suck air through and to blow into. We talk about the 'green, yellow, and red' zones of asthma and what to do for each. At home, epinephrine injections are a thing of the past. The medical breakthrough that allowed asthma treatment to come out of the dark ages was the inhaled steroid.

If asthma treatment were confectionary science, inhaled steroids would be Sir Isaac Newton. Newton may be best known as the brilliant scientist who first explained gravity and provided a theory to explain the motion of the planets. But his big contribution to confectionary science was figuring out how to stuff fruit inside a cake pastry, thereby taking fig farming from a fringe middle eastern niche into a global giant of an industry. Before Newton, fruit and cake were served on separate platters. After Newton's breakthrough, people could either buy one less serving platter or serve other snack items like nuts! It was liberating! Party hosting was never the same.

Inhaled steroids had the same liberating effect on asthma treatment. No longer would asthmatics have to undergo painful injections. They could prevent bad asthma attacks in the first place. The occasional exposure to a trigger didn't mean a life-threatening asthma attack anymore and asthmatics could expand their repertoire of physical activity.

Inhaled steroids accomplish all these magical things by treating the root problem in asthma—inflammation. If asthma were candy, inflammation would be sugar. Without sugar, there can be no candy. (Oh, sure, there's sugar-free candy, but that's the work of aliens!) So using an inhaled steroid is like stealing sugar from a candy maker. When inhaled steroids get into the lungs, they penetrate the airways and take away the inflammation (sugar) thereby preventing the airways from making asthma (candy). The result is patients controlling the disease instead of the disease controlling patients.

Nowadays, inhaled steroids come in powders, puffers, and liquids that can be put into machines that turn them into steam. They come in circular and cylindrical containers with knobs, levers, and counters, and in all the colors of the rainbow, so there can be no excuses. Every asthmatic, except the ones with the mildest forms, should be using an inhaled steroid.

An important distinction needs to be made between inhaled steroids and steroid pills. Steroid pills have a lot of very dangerous side effects, such as raising blood pressure and blood sugar, increasing weight, and increasing risk of stroke. Steroid pills cause these side effects because they enter the blood stream and disrupt the hormonal balance in the body. Inhaled steroids work only in the lungs. They do not enter the blood stream and therefore leave the body's natural hormonal balance untouched. They are *very* considerate that way.

So the next time we're enjoying a fruit-filled pastry or the effects of the earth's gravity, let's take a moment to thank the inhaled steroids. Thanks to them, the lives of asthmatics are closer to that of non-asthmatics than ever before. In fact, many people only find out that a friend has asthma after peering in their medicine cabinet. Medicine may be more complicated today, but it has also given us better treatment options. So I can do my paperwork, resting assured that, nowadays, I can better treat my patients' asthma—as well as my own.

Zoster's on the Roster— Permanently

Like an eclipse that blots out the sun, the red stripe creeps along its dermatomal path, blanketing the area already scouted by the red bumps. But the color is the least of the patient's worries because by now, the pain has taken hold and it's unlike any other. It's an out-of-this-world kind of pain. It's the kind of biblical pain that God inflicts on infidels—the really infidelious ones. It's 'lancing', 'shearing', 'searing' and all around 'owie!' *This* is shingles.

In medical school, the rash of shingles, aka 'Zoster', is described as ' . . . dew drops on a rose petal.' When I first read that description (having never seen an actual case of shingles in my life), it sounded like a rather pleasant thing. I pictured early mornings out in a garden with a running stream, some string music in the background, wine and cheese, and an ethnic woman in an ethnic outfit dancing an enticing ethnic dance that involves provocative use of the shoulders and wrists. (It's not that I had a particularly active imagination in medical school; it's just that the everyday drudgery and humiliation made me take refuge in my own special place(s), and it didn't take much to send me soaring. Those of you who watch the show *Scrubs* know what I'm talking about. But I digress.)

But the reality of Zoster is quite different. It is most certainly no walk in the park. It is no picnic, either. There's no wine, no cheese, and certainly no ethnic music nor dancing.

Zoster gets its name from the virus that causes it: Varicella Zoster Virus (VZV). This is the same virus that causes chicken pox.

As it turns out, getting the chicken pox is like head-butting someone in the World Cup Final. No matter what else you accomplish, or how many charity matches you set up, you will always be known as 'the head-butt guy'. Chicken pox has that same kind of permanence.

When people get chicken pox and recover from it, the virus never leaves the body. It simply goes into hiding. Specifically, it hides in the nerves. It brings a small hibachi, some lawn chairs, a few books and a laptop. And it just hangs out. Every once in a while, it'll peek its head out of the tent to see if the white blood cells are still patrolling the area. And if they are, it goes back into the tent and picks off where it left off in its 'My Space' blog.

But if it ever peeks its head out and notices the white blood cells fatigued or distracted by another infection, it decides to go for an outing. It hops on a nerve and rides it all the way to the end—at the skin. It opens small holes in the form of blisters and starts dumping out copies of itself. When the job is done, it closes up shop in the form of scabs on the blisters and goes back home. Perhaps it enjoys some finely aged liquor and relishes in a job well done.

If only that were the end of the story.

The poor nerve cell that has just been ridden by the Zoster virus sometimes gets so shocked by what has just happened that it remains on edge. It continues to send signals of pain long after the virus has gone. Much like how, after finding a flea on the cat, I start seeing little jumping black specks everywhere, the nerve cell in question screams 'pain!' even with things that aren't normally painful, such as touch, temperature and pressure.

That is the real woe of Zoster, because this pain can last a while. It is called 'neuralgia': 'neur-' meaning nerve and '-algia' meaning pain.

So beware ye elderly who have had chicken pox and thought it gone. The chicken pox remaineth. Your best bet is to stay healthy, consider a vaccine if you're over 60 (yes, we do have one now), and see your doctor soon if the symptoms develop. The sooner treatment is started, the more effective it is at sending the virus back into hiding and calming the nerve.

The Decade in Review

I heard from someone that the reason antibiotics are administered in ten-day courses is because that's how many fingers people have. Maybe that's how the metric system came into being: the French were tired of having to rely on passersby's appendages so they used a system based on divisions of ten. So ten years into not only the new decade or the new century, but the new *millennium*, it's natural to want to reflect on the events of the last decade.

To compile a comprehensive list of noteworthy health-related events of the last ten years would be like trying to compress the entire J.R.R. Tolkien catalog of Hobbit-related novels into motion pictures, i.e., something that only the truly talented can do. Instead, I offer my own abridged version of the last decade in health.

The decade got off to quite an exciting start with anthrax attacks through the mail. I'm assuming the responsible parties had to resort to "snail mail" after their email accounts failed to attach the white powder they had stuffed into their computers' USB ports. Politicians, high profile people, and low profile people with over-sized self-regard started getting nervous about opening their mail for fear of finding it laced with white powder. The trend was a ray of hope for the otherwise down-trodden Royal Food-Tasters lobby. This was their chance for employment in the modern world! Instead of tasting food for Royalty to check for poison, they could open people's mail to check for anthrax! But alas, it did not last.

Just as things were beginning to normalize, along came the Avian Flu. Suddenly, Asian poultry was getting a lot of press time, but not without a cost. At the slightest human cough, hordes of chickens, ducks, and geese were rounded up and slaughtered. Everyone was so nervous about catching bird flu that no one even thought about seizing the opportunity to make the world's largest chicken fajita! The key event everyone watched for with baited breath was human-to-human transmission of the virus. Luckily for Kevin Bacon, there was never more than one degree of human-to-human transmission and soon the rest of the world lost interest.

The last decade also gave us some medical breakthroughs. We got a new vaccine to prevent cervical cancer in women. It was, ideally, to be administered before girls became sexually active. Most doctors started administering it with the tetanus booster at the twelve-year old physical. This brought about many awkward moments in a pre-teen's health visit where the doctor would discuss the vaccine and how cervical cancer was caused by a virus that is transmitted through sex, and the pre-teen and accompanying parent would be mortified at the thought. Fortunately, the shot was so painful that it gave parents and pre-teens something to talk about on the car ride home.

Vaccine manufacturers also came out with a vaccine for seniors: the shingles vaccine. This was for anyone over the age of sixty who, for whatever reason, did not care to have excruciating nerve pain that lasted for months and wreaked havoc on their daily lives. But this vaccine wasn't without its share of pain, either. Except that, in this case, the pain was financial. Insurance companies batted their eyelashes and turned away when it came time to reimbursing physicians for the vaccine. So physicians did not take it upon themselves to purchase and store the vaccine. That's when the pharmacies stepped in to fill the void. Anyone who wanted a shingles vaccine had to get a prescription from their doctor, find a pharmacy that would fill it, hope the insurance would pay for it, then quickly return the vaccine to the doctor's office to be injected into them before the vaccine thawed, hoping that the stress of the ordeal itself wouldn't give them a case of shingles.

The 21st century also started us off with an official, honest-to-goodness pandemic. The novel H1N1, aka 'H1N1', aka 'swine flu', aka 'hand sanitizer baths for everybody', rose from humble beginnings in Mexico to infect the world. Then the race was on to contain the disease while trying to find a vaccine. Public health authorities were kind enough to issue guidelines as to who should be treated with anti-flu medications. Doctors were kind enough to write prescriptions, when appropriate. And patients spent the rest of the flu season going from pharmacy to pharmacy, searching for the universally unavailable drug, ensuring that pharmacy staff all over town were amply exposed to the virus.

Fortunately, public education on how to prevent the spread of the disease and vaccination against H1N1 worked well enough to keep the pandemic from truly wreaking havoc on the world.

The H1N1 virus is still with us. It's just taking some time off, probably relaxing on a beach somewhere. I'm sure it'll be back during cold and flu season.

Prior to the H1N1 excitement, resistant Staph, code name MRSA, tried to make a name for itself. Initially, there was much concern about a super bug that was resistant to all but one or two antibiotics. But then, when all it did was cause people boils and impetigo, the excitement quickly waned.

As public excitement ebbed and flowed over these various infections and vaccines, America's stalwarts of chronic disease—obesity, diabetes, high blood pressure, high cholesterol and heart disease—tried to keep a low profile and go unnoticed. And their strategy was brilliant! They set out to make themselves so prominent that people would actually not notice them—like cloudy days in Seattle. They walked around pointing out various new infections and gasping in an overly exaggerated manner. They feigned anger and fear. They argued that *they* didn't cause people to feel bad! They were just slow moving diseases! There was no need for alarm. They urged us to take care of these more pressing illnesses first.

And things were working out pretty well for them almost until the end of this decade, when the newly elected First Lady noticed childhood obesity hiding in a crowd with its beanie pulled down low, pretending to listen to its iPod, and she decided to take action.

This was bad news for the rest of America's reliable chronic diseases. Studies had shown that obese children grew up to become obese adults. So by reducing childhood obesity, it stood to reason that, eventually, there would be less adult obesity. But that could be just the beginning! If there were less adult obesity, that could reduce diabetes, high cholesterol, high blood pressure, heart disease, arthritis, and certain cancers, just to name a few. This approach could very well cripple America's chronic disease industry! Who, then, will take on the mantle of hosting these chronic diseases??? China???

So as we start the new decade, one can't help but wonder what new and exciting health-related events await us. What exotic or well-known-but-mutated disease will test our collective response? What new breakthroughs in prevention and treatment await us? Will we truly derail any of our blue chip diseases? Will we have enough song-and-dance-based reality shows to get us through? I don't know about you, but I can't wait to find out!

www.ingramcontent.com/pod-product-compliance
Lightning Source LLC
Chambersburg PA
CBHW031832170526
45157CB00001B/270